# IT'S YOUR BODY

# IT'S YOUR BODY

## *MOVE IT, LOVE IT, LIVE*

## VANESSA BOGENHOLM

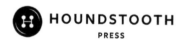

## HOUNDSTOOTH
### PRESS

IT'S YOUR BODY
*Move It, Love It, Live*

ISBN   978-1-5445-2261-6   *Hardcover*
       978-1-5445-2260-9   *Paperback*
       978-1-5445-2259-3   *Ebook*
       978-1-5445-2262-3   *Audiobook*

*This book is dedicated to my dear friend Jack.
Jack was the first client I helped get out of a
wheelchair, stand up, and walk with a walker.
He was the grandfather I never had, and I miss
him every day. Rest in peace, my friend, and yes,
I am staying out of the bars, kind of, sometimes.*

# CONTENTS

*PART 1*

## DO I REALLY THINK YOU NEED TO READ ANOTHER FITNESS BOOK? NOPE, BUT THIS ONE IS COMPLETELY DIFFERENT.

*Chapter 1:* Why Did I Write This Book?   **3**

*Chapter 2:* Admit to Yourself You Want to Get Healthy   **9**

*Chapter 3:* I've Been Where You Are   **19**

*PART 2*

## LIVING IN YOUR BODY

*Chapter 4:* My Personal Pain   **43**

*Chapter 5:* Evaluating Your Own Pain   **49**

*Chapter 6:* Honesty Is Hard. Being Human is Hard.   **61**

*Chapter 7:* Understand What Your Body Needs   **67**

*Chapter 8:* Let's Start Moving!   **83**

# EXERCISES

Walking **90**

Weight and Leg Extensions **92**

Step-Ups **94**

Standing up without Using Your Arms **96**

Sit-Ups **98**

Straight Leg Raise **100**

Core Balance with a Twist **102**

Sit-up with a Twist, Legs Straight **104**

Running **106**

Push-Ups **108**

Push-up to Leg Extension **110**

Modified Dead Bug **112**

Lunges **114**

Arm Extensions **116**

Bicep Curl and Shoulder Push **118**

Jumping **120**

Stretches **122**

Exercise Everywhere **124**

PART 3

# LET'S MEET SOME REAL PEOPLE

*Chapter 9:* People Are Different. My Approaches Are Different Too. **129**

*Chapter 10:* How I Approach Working with a New Client **133**

*Chapter 11:* Obesity: What It Really Is and How Much It Affects a Person's Life **145**

*Chapter 12:* Meet Some of My (Formerly) Obese Clients   **151**

*Chapter 13:* Workouts and Lifestyle Changes
for Overweight/Obese Clients   **169**

*Chapter 14:* Dad Bods and the Constantly Sitting Man   **177**

*Chapter 15:* Workouts and Lifestyle Changes
for Middle-Aged Men   **193**

*Chapter 16:* Women 40–70 Can Still Look
Hot and Be Incredible!   **199**

*Chapter 17:* Helping Women Get the Bodies
They Want and Deserve   **211**

*Chapter 18:* Teenagers, Athletic and Not:
Think Fitness, Not Sports   **217**

*Chapter 19:* Lifelong Movement and Good Eating
Habits for Soon-to-Be Adults   **233**

*Chapter 20:* Over 70: "Never Done It,"
"It's Too Hard," "My Body's Shot."   **239**

*Chapter 21:* Getting People over 70 to Move   **251**

*Chapter 22:* Take Your First Step: Set Achievable Goals   **253**

*Chapter 23:* Stay Motivated for Life   **257**

Acknowledgements   **261**
About the Author   **263**

# PART 1

*DO I REALLY THINK YOU NEED TO READ ANOTHER FITNESS BOOK?*

# NOPE, BUT THIS ONE IS COMPLETELY DIFFERENT.

# CHAPTER 1

# WHY DID I WRITE THIS BOOK?

*I* went to the grocery store one evening after seeing ten personal training clients. I was physically and emotionally tired past the point of complete exhaustion. As I was shopping, I had the feeling someone was following me around the grocery store. In the produce section, I saw a woman a little too close on my right side. When I looked in her direction, she was staring directly at my face. In the fish section, she was standing right behind me. In the bread section, she was still right behind me. I thought I was being paranoid until I saw her again to my left going down another aisle and glancing away from me when I looked in her direction.

Before I could think too much about her, I ran into a friend, and we started to have a conversation about my marathon training and overall running for the year. We also chatted about other aspects of our lives. We laughed together about the glory of going through the pain of running and finding happiness with our running and in our lives. The mystery woman stood right across from us and was listening to our entire conversation. After I hugged my friend goodbye, I couldn't stand it anymore. "I'm sorry—do we know each other?" I asked the woman in an aggravated voice.

"No, I am sorry," she said. "You just look so incredibly happy and fit. I just was—well, I wouldn't even know what to do with most of the stuff in your shopping cart. I heard you are a runner. You look very inspirational." She put her head down, so she wouldn't have to look me in the eye while she was speaking to me.

I looked in her grocery cart, filled with boxes of processed foods, frozen entrees, and sugary desserts, including Twinkies. I had always wondered if there was even any real food in a Twinkie. I looked at my cart, filled with fresh vegetables and fruit, still warm bakery bread, and a piece of salmon rounding out my cart for my dinner that evening.

"I am a personal trainer. I have my own fitness studio in San Jose," I responded, smiling and standing just a little bit taller, overly proud of myself and my professional accomplishments.

"I bet you are expensive," she responded. "I could never afford someone like you to help me."

This time I dropped my eyes, so I didn't have to look at the woman. Because she was right: I am expensive. I charge clients by the hour, and most clients see me for either two or three hours every week. My schedule has been full for many years, and the majority of my clients have been with me for more than four years. The cost of having me as a personal trainer in a private studio costs thousands of dollars per year for each client.

I could never have afforded a personal trainer like me when I was unathletic and overweight as a child. I didn't even know personal trainers existed when I was overweight in the late 1970s and early 1980s. I could have used guidance on my fitness journey back when I first started losing weight and caring about my body as a teenager. I had to learn everything out of books from the library or from people I met who gave me free advice. The books I read pushed me in the right direction, but I never saw someone like me in those books. I never saw a sad, overweight child (or angry, overweight adult) who had no clue how to move their bodies—in any book I read. I still don't see those kinds of books written now. I never see the pain, the tears, and the frustration everyone feels as they try to change their bodies every day in my studio. This isn't just physical pain but emotional pain and frustration.

I thanked the woman for the compliments and wished her well as I started to leave the grocery store. Then I felt very conflicted and ran after her. "Just walk ten minutes a day. That will be a great start for you. When you want to eat junk food, or any processed food, just drink a full glass of water first. Maybe two glasses. Drink warm water or tea before dinner. Something warm in your stomach helps ease the feeling of hunger. Dehydration causes us to feel hungry too. These little lifestyle changes can do wonders." I put on a very forced smile. She smiled as a response to this barrage of suggestions, but I knew she didn't listen to any of the words I had just thrown at her. I could tell she felt the things I suggested were just beyond her ability.

I drove home feeling like I had failed this woman horribly. Of course, I was proud of myself for building a business that helped people reach their health goals and become happier in life. But I wanted to reach more people with my personal training methods and strategies. The guilt of only being available to people with larger sums of disposable income was getting to me. I didn't want to be a personal trainer only for the rich. I wanted to touch people's lives and help them believe they could change their bodies and their minds.

So, why didn't I write that book with the honest truth about how people start getting fit and feeling better about their health and bodies? A book of truth and inspiration for everyone to enjoy their bodies. The type of book that would have helped me so much when I was the fat, sad, angry child stuck in a body that felt out of control. Those thoughts of writing this book plagued me on the drive home from the grocery store and in the upcoming weeks.

This book, *It's Your Body: Move It, Love It, Live*, is going to be completely different from any fitness book you have ever read.

This book is about how real people change their bodies for the better. Real people who can't get out of a wheelchair. Real people who need to lose one hundred pounds or more. Teenagers who have never participated in sports. Middle-aged men who are so out of shape and unhealthy, they are taking six or more prescription pills a day. Women who can't believe their bodies are sagging this badly in their forties.

You will join my clients and me on their fitness journeys, and I hope they inspire you to start your own. I feel grateful I have been able to help so many people move forward with their bodies. Now I want to help you without the expense of seeing me in person.

In this book, I will discuss the reality of what I see every day in my fitness studio. The good, positive changes. The bad, including the pain and the failures. You will meet amazing people that changed not just their physical bodies but also their mental attitudes.

I will give you simple, daily tasks to do to improve your body. Don't expect anything extreme, and realize this transformation will take time.

I hope this book will inspire you to want a healthier body that you can enjoy without pain. I want you to do the things with your body you have always dreamed of: Run your first 5K. Play football with your grandchildren. Look hot in that little black dress at the company dinner. Easily get out of a chair or the bathtub. We are all unique and have different motivations in life. I want to help you find your inspiration for change.

This book is for everyone who has tried to lose weight, exercise more, and feel comfortable in their bodies. I want you to be inspired to be the best you can be.

Join me on this journey to feeling better through everyday exercise and dealing with food issues and pain management. Let's move toward a body you can love and be proud to live in.

# CHAPTER 2

# ADMIT TO YOURSELF YOU WANT TO GET HEALTHY

A dmit it: you are reading this book because you want the motivation to get healthy and feel better. You just don't know how to, no matter how many times you have dedicated yourself to changing your exercise and eating patterns. Let's be honest: change is physically and mentally challenging for everyone.

In this book, I will address the reality of our human bodies: the physical and mental pains of obesity, the difficulty and embarrassment of people who have never worked out, the injuries and illnesses normal people mask with over-the-counter and prescription pills, and noncommittal physical activity. Our bodies were made to move.

Human beings shouldn't be embarrassed as they try to make their bodies the best they can, but almost all of my clients are embarrassed when they start working out with me. A common theme is they think they should be better, move better, look better, and feel better. Most clients are embarrassed they have become so overweight—"Why can't I exercise for more than a minute without being out of breath?" and "I don't understand why I'm in constant pain." It doesn't matter to me where a client starts. What matters is their willingness to start moving forward to a better body.

As I approached writing a book about what I do with the people who walk through my fitness studio door every week, I needed to think about how I help my personal training clients. Everyone comes to me wanting to "get fit and feel better physically in their own bodies," but what does that mean? For some, it means losing weight; for some, it's cutting sugar out of their diets, so their brains feel better and their bodies become smaller; for others, it's moving around through exercise, so their joints feel better; for still others, it's to have better lung capacity and heart health. No two people whom I have worked with have ever come to me for the same reasons. As a client becomes more comfortable with me, they tell me their reasons evolve and change.

A common question from a new client is, "What kind of exercises are we going to do?" I usually just smile and start some kind of warm-up exercise because, honestly, I don't know. I need to see what shape their bodies are in to start. I need to observe how crooked their bodies might be, where they might have injuries, how much pain they are in, and the big one: how scared they are of working out and moving their bodies. Because of remembered pain, many people are scared to try to move their bodies. Our brains trick us every day into staying the way we are, no matter how hard we want to change.

Mostly, when I first start working with a new client, I need to listen. I need to listen to the person they are, what their daily activity looks like, what their home and work life entails, who they want to be, and I need to figure out how to help them get to the place they want to be, even if that place seems so out of reach to them. I also need to get them to listen to themselves and their bodies, not just tell me about them.

Then, I make a plan. It's a plan consisting of thoughts I might write down immediately but not necessarily share with the client all at once. Honestly, it takes about two months working with a client until I figure out how to work them out and get to the direction we will go through together.

This book is very different than what you currently see in the fitness marketplace. Now there are millions of health and fitness books with ridiculous crash and fad diets: shake diets, grapefruit diets, intermittent fasting, diets based on your blood type, and of course, vegan and keto. There are even more books with exercise programs that say things like, "Work out just ten minutes a day!" and "Forty-five minutes a day to get beautiful abs," and who can forget the shake weight, thigh master, etc.? There are tons of at-home equipment, from expensive exercise bikes to straps you hang on a doorknob. I guess those diets and gadgets work for some people to lose weight and get fit, but for how many people? So, what is actually missing from all of that equipment and those books, videos, blogs, etc.? I mean, have you ever met a real human being who got fit and stayed healthy from a cabbage diet and a shake weight at home on their exercise bike?

> *The missing link is the respect for*
> *your body and the motivation to take*
> *care of your body to feel better.*

There is always that overly fit person at work that will swear they lost ten pounds in a week on a juice cleanse, and you should too. "Here, I have a custom link just for you!" Did they tell you that, by getting you signed up for the crazy diet, they would get their crazy disgusting-tasting green juice for free? It's kind of the new marketing scheme: "share a sale" and ambassadorships are what these sales techniques are called in the marketing world. Or, maybe, it was some new amazing probiotics your friend is pushing on you with no medical data whatsoever, saying they'll clean out your colon because, obviously, you aren't fat because you eat too much of the wrong kinds of food and don't move your body. No, instead, you are just backed up with partially decomposed food, making your stomach and intestines stick out. Yuck.

So, how does the average person who wants to get fit and has a few pounds to lose or joints that hurt start this fitness journey? Like you. How about the post office worker who walks all day and carries a bag on only the right side of her body, so her shoulders and back are very crooked, or the tech guy at his desk all day with a rounded back and his neck sticking forward? How about the person who has a job that takes up forty to sixty desk hours plus ten hours of commute times a week? How about the family that can't take more than fifteen minutes to make dinner and eats dinner while standing up over the kitchen sink or in front of the computer while talking and texting to other people, ignoring the family members in the same room.

Maybe your doctor prescribed you two to three—or even six or more—drugs a day for all kinds of ailments, and you can't sleep (because you are over forty-five years old and exhausted all the time). How do you get fit and healthy when you are too tired for exercise and feel sick most of the time? How does anyone? And if you get fit, how do you stay fit and healthy for the rest of your life? Is it even possible?

Our brains can be our own worst enemy. Our thoughts can sabotage us.

"What is wrong with me? Why does everyone else lose twenty pounds a month on this new fad diet/exercise program and not me? In fact, why did I actually gain weight after I joined the gym or started a running program? And why can't I ever stick to a program for more than a week? Am I just a weak person?"

"It must be just the way I am supposed to be. My body is comfortable at this weight," we rationalize with ourselves.

We tell ourselves this is fine and accept that we are "just a little overweight" and hurt and taking lots of pills because "well, everyone else I hang out with is overweight and in pain, and the doctor said I need to take these pills, so I take them."

And the most common rationalization I hear: "I am not as fat or out of shape as that guy!" That guy could be anyone—a stranger at the grocery store, someone at work, a family member. We compare ourselves to other human beings to prop up our own fragile egos.

Now we go to the "body acceptance" kick we see now on social media and in all kinds of magazine and newspaper publications. No reason to get fit and healthy. It is perfectly okay to be overweight and out of shape; it is normal. Americans are just bigger now. We physically move less in modern society. Clothing companies have increased their sizes to fit American bodies. This up in size is referred to as "vanity" sizing. Women feel better about themselves because even though the scale and the mirror tell them they have gained weight, they bought a smaller pant size, so they feel good about themselves and buy more clothes. Instagram tells me it is okay to be fat—I can still be sexy. I see fat women in bikinis, and being fat is easier anyway, isn't it? More self-rationalization.

But deep down, you know you are overweight and not taking care of your body, and you don't feel good about it. Your body hurts all the time, even when you roll over in bed onto that shoulder and hip that seems to be in constant pain. You want to look and feel better emotionally, too, not just physically. You don't even know now if you are in more physical pain or mental pain, or which pain came first. You are lost in indecision and lack motivation, and the last thing you want to do is try another exercise and diet program and have it fail.

Being overweight and out of shape isn't the easier option, though. Being overweight and not exercising and moving these bodies we live in is physically painful and emotionally depressing. Your knees hurt, your back hurts, and to fit into an airplane seat is just plain embarrassing. Let's not even talk about that chair you broke at your friend's house at the party or that the toilet that needs to be replaced in your home because you broke that also from weighing too much for it to handle.

I know, and I understand. I was obese as a child. My stomach was so large and stuck out over my feet, so I couldn't see my shoes. I didn't even know I was fat until a ten-year-old classmate told me I was fat. It was just the way it was for my life as a child and in my family. We were all fat, and no one in my family exercised. After this classmate told me I was fat, I did all those crazy diets and fad exercise programs as a child to try and lose the weight. I bought the pills at the drugstore that guaranteed I would lose ten pounds a week. I watched the videos with overly fit movie stars like Jane Fonda jumping around in her leg warmers. I watched Jack LaLanne on TV exercising with a chair, tried to not eat solid foods (that lasted six hours), and failed miserably from those so-called "diets" and exercise kicks that would last less than a week. I stayed fat as a child for four more years after that girl told me I was fat, though I desperately searched for and tried weight-loss techniques. I gave up every time.

I have heard my clients and many acquaintances talk about their failures with long-term weight loss and exercise programs. We have all watched celebrities go up and down with their weight and wellness also.

If the rich and famous, who have more than enough money and people to help them—chefs, personal trainers, nutritionists, hypnotherapists, and the time to dedicate to their bodies and health—can't stick to a diet and exercise program, how is the average person like you going to do it? Is it even possible for you to lose weight and get healthy?

Here is the first big revelation.

*You need to admit to yourself you want a better body.*

You need to admit you want to feel better and get healthy. This mental shift will take some serious change and a commitment on your part.

Admit to yourself that getting healthy doesn't start with just a diet, an exercise class once a week, drinking more water, shaking around that shake weight, and blaming your parents for your fat genes and lack of exercise...

*No, it starts with you admitting you have a problem, a serious one. Admit that you want to get fit and feel better. Emotionally commit to this new lifestyle choice. Because that is what "this" really is: a new lifestyle choice.* **A healthier new life is your choice.**

I am not saying losing one hundred pounds, not eating cheeseburgers, passing on the office donuts, getting those biceps noticed by the cute office girl, and running your first 5K will be easy with arthritis in those knee joints. You make a mental decision, and—poof!—all these great things happen. It is not easy. In fact, this will probably be the hardest thing you will ever do in your life. But in the end, you will get a body you can love and appreciate. The body you deserve.

These lifestyle changes will be tough, physically and emotionally, and you will cry and scream and get mad and disappointed and want to give up numerous times. Sometimes you will give up many times in a single day, or a single hour.

But when you finally realize you have control over your body, with your mind and your decisions, you will be happier than you ever dreamed of and will be content and able to move forward with the new fitter lifestyle that will bring you happiness. Not just physical happiness but emotional happiness too.

# CHAPTER 3

# I'VE BEEN
# WHERE YOU ARE

My name is Vanessa Bogenholm, and I am the most un-athletic person you will ever meet. I grew up embarrassingly poor. I spent most of my childhood years in a single-wide mobile home with my fat father. My father had that big belly hanging over his belt—the kind of hard, visceral fat belly commonly referred to as "beer belly"—so he couldn't see his shoes. My father smoked Lark Long cigarettes that stained not just his teeth but the kitchen ceiling yellow. He drank heavily every day cheap Lucky Store brand vodka or Lucky Lager beer. My father couldn't keep a job over two months because he always thought he was smarter than his bosses.

My mother went to her federal employee job Monday through Friday, 9:00 a.m. to 5:00 p.m., figuring out how much overtime she could accumulate when the government needed real work to be done. She ordered helicopter parts for the National Guard, so wars were good for her vacation pay. My mother looked out the kitchen window at home, ignoring what was happening in her own home with her family. Starting at fourteen, my brother was an on-again-off-again convict, imprisoned for selling drugs, robbery, pimping, or violence—or, sometimes, all of these crimes rolled together. Eventually, my brother did long prison stints for armed robbery and murder.

My sister got out of the house right at sixteen years old to go to college and moved away from the chaos that was our home. I don't blame her. She had to get out to save herself. Alone as a child, I read about life in library books and sought comfort from my dogs, my ever-loving and great lifelong companions.

Children are cruel, but their meanness moved me in the right direction. As twisted as it is, I am grateful for their honesty. When I was ten years old, I attended a small Catholic grade school in Santa Maria, CA. I was the new kid at this school with twenty-eight students in the class. My parents had moved us to Santa Maria from the Los Angeles area after my father had used a shotgun to blow up our front porch in Lakewood, CA, when two guys came looking for my brother. My brother had recently been arrested and was in jail. The guys wanted money my brother owed them from a drug deal. My father shot at them with a shotgun, so the men left in a hurry. He missed them but damaged our front porch. No one called the police. I guess, in our neighborhood, gunshots were common.

The next day after the shooting, I showed my dad the drawer full of torn-up cigarettes in my brother's room. It was marijuana, but I had no idea. After seeing this, my father felt we—my mother, him, and me—needed a fresh start in a small town. He literally chose Santa Maria off a Triple-A map laid out on the kitchen table the next evening after dinner. We moved from Lakewood to Santa Maria within two months. One of those months we spent living in a dive motel where I played in the dumpster on crushed cardboard boxes. I thought living in the motel was fun. I didn't care about moving. I didn't have any friends or activities I was leaving behind in Los Angeles.

At lunchtime on a Thursday at St. Mary's Grade School—I can still remember even what day of the week it was—I unpacked the lunch my mother had made for me. My mother always packed a frozen cola in my lunch, wrapped in aluminum foil to keep it cold until lunchtime. I had been at this new school, in this new town, for about a month.

The popular girl with boobs (remember, we were in the fifth grade, so all of us were ten or eleven years old) and pretty, shiny hair said to me, "You know drinking a Coke every day is bad for you. That's why you're fat." I didn't speak back to her; I kept my head down and stared at my lunch. I didn't know I was fat. Honestly. No one had ever told me before that I was fat. I just thought I was the big girl—big-boned or whatever. Big for my age. That was why girl's clothes didn't fit me, why I had to shop in the boy's section for size eighteen Husky Jeans from Montgomery Ward and Sears.

Then, another pretty popular girl said to me, *"You can eat your lunch with us, but you can't play with us."* She giggled and turned to the other five girls to share the joke with them. That statement will forever be burned into my brain. I got up from the school bench next to the chain-link fence and threw away my lunch. I went and sat on the cement walkway by the bathrooms, down a hallway, away from the other kids. No one followed me. No fellow students, not the adult playground monitor. No one cared about the fat new girl.

I tried to play sports in grade school and middle school, but I was overweight and uncoordinated. I couldn't shoot a basketball and was always the last to be picked on the softball team because I always struck out. I needed glasses for horrible astigmatism, but my parents couldn't afford the cost of the glasses and would just tell me to sit in the front of the class closer to the board so I could see the day's lessons.

But, man, did those grade school boys throw the ball hard at me during Dodge ball. I was too heavy to move fast enough to get out of the way. I can still hear the boys' laughter and remember every one of the boys' faces. Dodge ball on those grade school playgrounds made me hate any sport with a ball. (Dodge ball should be illegal on all school grounds, in my opinion.)

I spent most of my time outside of school reading and eating large amounts of candy. This candy was a treat that I got from my parents as a child. We would go to the Sears Department Store and spend ten dollars at the candy counter. Sears back then had these candy counters with big glass boxes and scoops. This candy was my friend. It made my brain feel good, and I would shove the sugar into my mouth as fast as I could. I never remember the two to three pounds of candy lasting me more than a day.

My mother was a horrible cook. I ate frozen toaster waffles for breakfast, white-bread fried bologna sandwiches drenched in Mayonnaise with BBQ chips for lunch, and a hunk of meat and potatoes for dinner with sliced white bread smeared with bright yellow margarine that looked like it had been hit by a nuclear reactor.

I never remember going to a doctor (except to a dentist, once, where I learned I had fourteen cavities as a seven- or eight-year-old child).

I had asthma (I think because of my father's smoking). I had over-the-counter Primatene Mist inhalers for my breathing issues, just like my father used at the kitchen table every morning as he coughed his guts out while he smoked his cigarettes and drank coffee. I also had severe allergies, hay fever, that I took over-the-counter pills for that made me sleepy. I look stoned in class most of the time from those allergy pills.

But the summer before high school, that all changed.

Santa Maria was a basketball town. My mother was hoping I would play basketball in high school even though I never did an entire season in junior high basketball. In junior high, we had a coach that yelled all the time. He would yell so much at us young girls in games he would spit as he yelled at you. I heard enough yelling at home and didn't want to hear it in school activities too. I quit the junior high school basketball team one day after the coach screamed at us during a game. When I quit the team, no one, not the players or the coach, even asked me why. The coach just took my uniform. I guess I wasn't needed or wanted and wouldn't be missed on the basketball team.

*This response of not even asking me why I was quitting by the junior high basketball coach taught me quitting was okay when something wasn't fun or I wasn't good at it.*

I went to a basketball camp at my new high school during the summer before high school started. When we ran sprints across the gym and back, I was always the slowest girl out there. I had no vertical jump. Literally. My shoes didn't come off the floor. I had never learned how to shoot a basketball properly, so that was out too. I mean, I was two hundred pounds and shot granny-goose style—you know, ball underhand between your legs. I remember my "friends" laughing at me because I was so bad. Coach Hearn, at St. Joseph High School in Orcutt, CA, was an incredibly nice person. He didn't say I was fat, or slow, or uncoordinated. He never said anything negative to me.

What Coach Hearn did say was, "Vanessa, you probably want to get fit before basketball season starts." This was the summer of 1980, two months before my fourteenth birthday. I had just started a job at the mall, selling leather shoes at Western Boots. The owner of the store I worked in also owned the Footlocker in the same mall.

I may have been overweight, unathletic, and didn't have any friends, but I wasn't lazy and wanted to get out of that single wide mobile home we lived in. I was working to buy a real house for my mom and me, so I could get a dog. Getting a dog was my biggest motivation. I hadn't had a dog in four years since we moved to Santa Maria after my brother's arrest. At my first job at the age of ten, I cleaned horse stables, then I worked at the Fairgrounds at the age of thirteen, and by this point, at fourteen, I worked thirty hours a week in a mall. I worked and saved my money for three and a half years before I started high school to buy a real home and get out of the mobile home.

Frank Shorter, the man who started the American running craze in the 1970s, had been my hero for years. I watched the Olympic Marathon in 1972 when Mr. Shorter won the gold but lost the applause due to a cheater coming into the stadium and running right in front of him, confusing the audience. I watched the entire marathon again in 1976 when an East German drug user cheated and stole the gold from Mr. Shorter, who got the Silver Medal. Mr. Shorter could not compete in 1980 because the United States boycotted the Olympics due to politics. I was amazed a man who had missed his due glory over and over still had the internal strength of character to keep running over one hundred forty miles a week and training for decades. I wanted that character.

I never thought of being an athlete. Those people were special. And even though I thought I could never be a real athlete, I wanted the hard-working character of Mr. Shorter.

I went to the Santa Maria Public Library that Wednesday evening after the basketball camp with my father. I loved to escape in books, and this was the only thing my father and I shared: a love of reading and going to the library. I checked out every book on running they had, more than my arms could carry. My father never asked why I was checking out those running books. My father was too interested in his crime mysteries to notice the books I had chosen that evening. I remember the also overweight librarian smiling at me and letting me take home more than ten books, more than I was allowed to check out per week.

I felt something wet in my pants on the drive home from the library. Unbeknownst to me, I started my period that evening. I just thought I had a stomachache and was sick. The next morning, I realized what the blood was and told my mother. My father made jokes.

On my break the next day at work, I walked down to the Footlocker store. I knew my twenty percent discount worked there from the store's owner since he was also my employer. I picked out a pair of tan and brown Nikes for $19.99, bought the latest Runner's World Magazine, and went back to work at the Western Boot Store. For the rest of my work shift, I stared at those runners in the magazine, tiny shorts and defined leg muscles and agony on their faces. I was enthralled by their effort and drive. For the first time in my almost fourteen years, I dreamed of being an athlete, a runner.

I stayed up all night reading about famous runners, training schedules, food, and running form. I made a plan. Frank Shorter ran one hundred twenty to one hundred forty miles a week as most distance runners did according to the books, so I had to start tomorrow morning. I barely slept. I was so excited to start this new me and go running!

Being an early morning person, I got up, dressed in my old grey sweats, put on my new fancy Nike running shoes. I didn't say a word to my dad as he sat at the kitchen table, drinking his watered-down coffee, smoking Lark Long cigarettes, and reading a paperback western novel. I just went out of the front door to attack my run. My neighborhood had those yellow streetlights, and the morning mist was out. I put my head down and ran!

I counted twenty-three steps. My brain just automatically counts everything. I ran to the corner of the street is all, and we were the second house from the corner, so it wasn't very far. I seriously hurt! This wasn't the effortless Frank Shorter run; this was a fat girl with a heart about to explode. I couldn't catch my breath from my allergies and asthma and the secondhand smoke of my home. I sat on the corner under a streetlight and gave up.

*At this point, I believed I was the fat girl who could never be athletic. I completely gave up. Hot tears poured*

*from my eyes, and snot ran down my face as I sat on*
*that street corner under the yellow streetlamps.*

As I walked back home, I counted the twenty-three steps again.
I was utterly defeated, and this time, I cared that I was a loser
and a quitter. I realized why the other kids picked on me and
why I didn't have any friends. I was a sad, awful, fat girl with
no friends that no one wanted to be around. Nobody cares
about you when you don't care about yourself, Vanessa, I said
to myself.

As I went up to open the front door of my house, a real brand-
new house that I had bought for my parents that month, I
stopped. I had saved money for almost four years to buy a real
home for my mother and me. If I could work that hard to buy a
home, before the age of fourteen, why was I giving up on running and losing weight so quickly?

I decided not to give up this time. If I could run twenty-three
steps, what about twenty-four steps. Could I do just one more
step? I turned around and did even more than I had planned.
On my second attempt at running, I ran twenty-six steps! I ran
halfway around the corner. More than I even hoped for! How
about if I rested, caught my breath, then ran home? I did. I
caught my breath for a couple of minutes and then ran home as
my mother opened the front door and left for work.

"Vanessa, what are you doing outside?" my mother asked incred-
ulously. I didn't answer her. I just kept my head down, avoiding

her look. This running was only a promise to me, not to anyone else. No one was going to get why I was doing this or change my mind. I was going to be a runner!

It was 5:23 a.m., according to my Timex, and my life changed.

Every morning that summer, I got up between 4:30 a.m. and 4:45 a.m. and went out to run. I gave myself a visual, when I got tired or hurt, between five and ten steps ahead—a streetlight, a car, a tree, a driveway—that I would make myself run to, so I wouldn't give up. Some days I ran twice a day. I was alone with my Walkman, my Timex, my now-bloody socks, and a sense of accomplishment I had never had in my fourteen years of life. I wasn't doing this for anyone else but me.

I also started riding a moped that my drug-dealing brother had bought me for my birthday. I rode to the other end of town to the YMCA. The YMCA had a weight room, and you could use it for a quarter. I lifted weights at least twice a week. The running books called this lifting of weights "strength training," and all the articles said how important it was to be a good runner. I was always the only girl in the gym at the YMCA. I was also much younger than the men who worked out there. They were very nice to me and showed me how to use the machines and lift weights properly. They congratulated me when I could lift more weight or do more chin-ups. They were all encouraging and nonjudgmental. I had never met more encouraging people in my life. I liked these men who just wanted to help me and never made fun of me.

For the first time in my life, I felt like I belonged with these men working out. I was not made fun of as I was in school around my peers.

My mother came home one evening from work to our new home in mid-July at 5:15 p.m., her usual time. I was overly excited as I waited for her. I had been running for a little over a month. It was a week before my fourteenth birthday.

"Mom, can we go for a drive?" I asked.

She said, "Yes, of course," and asked, "Where?"

"Just out. I will tell you." My excitement was excruciating.

As we got into her car, I hit the button on the trip meter of her Cadillac. She didn't notice. "Turn right...turn left...go all the way into town...turn here." This drive was a circle all around the town of Santa Maria.

As we pulled into our driveway, I was full of excitement, "Mom! Mom! Tell me what the trip meter says!" I screamed.

"Vanessa, it says eleven miles. Did you actually run that far this morning?" she asked. This was the first time I remember my mother looking right at me in my eyes and not with pity or the drunken "don't bother me" look I was so used to seeing from her.

"Yes, oh yes, Mom! We have to go to Footlocker right now!"

My mother just figured I needed more socks or new running shoes, patted me on the shoulder (we weren't a hugging family), and drove me to the mall. We walked in, and I said "Hi" to the sales guys who knew me since we worked for the same man. The Footlocker employees were community college runners, all skinny and fit, always talking about running, injuries, and food. They asked me how my running was going, and I felt happy because I had something positive to talk about with these young, fit athletes. I felt like one of them when they asked me how my blisters were healing. We were soul mates in our love of running and taking care of our feet. I went to the bulletin board toward the back of the store and pulled off the paper entry for the ten-mile race from Guadalupe to Santa Maria that was to be held the next week during the Santa Barbara County Fair.

"Mom, I am under eighteen years old. I need you to sign this permission slip for me. I am entering a road race." She didn't ask any questions; instead, she signed the form and looked at the runners in the store in shock when they all wished me luck and high-fived me. "Go get 'em, Vanessa! Can't wait to see you finish that race," they all said to me, smiling. I wrote out a check to pay for the race. We went to the post office and mailed my race entry immediately.

I don't remember my mother speaking to me on the drive home. I don't think she or my father had paid much attention to my early morning running routine. They probably just thought it was a teenage phase. Something I would start and stop any day soon as I had done with so many things in my life. I told my mother I was going out for another run. I went out to rerun the eleven-mile course that day. This eleven-mile run was my regular running route for years. Kids in school would call me "the runner" as my nickname. Shop owners would come out and wave to me. It took me about an hour and thirty to thirty-five minutes every day, and my feet almost always fell asleep around mile eight. Running shoes were horrible back then, and my socks were a bloody mess all the time from constant blisters. But these runs made me happy. I was happy to be in charge of my body and accomplish something I thought was only a dream. I was running.

When I got home from that second run of the day, my mother had made pasta for dinner with fresh vegetables. She had followed a recipe out of *Runner's World* magazine. The magazine was sitting on the kitchen counter. We never discussed it, but after that day, she used *Runner's World* as her cookbook. She never made meat and potatoes for me again. She cooked healthy food, bleached out the bloodstains from my socks, and tied my feet to the bed when I cramped at night to show her silent, constant support for me.

I must point out this was 1980, and female runners were scarce. For this ten-mile race I had entered at the Santa Barbara County Fair, there were probably twenty men for every one woman. Anyone who lives around Santa Maria knows the winds of 3:00 p.m., and this race was an afternoon race right into that headwind. The men were very nice to this young girl running and very encouraging. I never remembered people smiling at me so much for just attempting something. I felt part of a large welcoming group of people, not alone. When I got tired at mile eight and slowed down, the men kept looking back and smiling as they passed me and saying things like, "Almost there! Good job! Just keep going! You look great!" Coming into the finish line at the Santa Barbara County Fairgrounds was everything to me. I had set a goal, an impossible goal for this fat girl—I mean, really, I had run ten miles in a real race—by taking just one more step, and I accomplished that goal. Two months earlier, I could only run twenty-three steps. I had pushed my body past its comfort zone and proved to myself I was in control of my body and I could do anything! As my mom drove me home after the race, I was so happy with my accomplishment. I made a silent goal to myself only—I'd run a marathon in one year.

Six weeks later, when high school started, I looked like a different person. I was 4′ taller, now almost 5′9″. I would finish out at 5′11″ and had dropped well over sixty pounds over the summer through my running and weightlifting. I didn't even know what cross-country was when I started high school. The coach had seen me running around town and asked why I didn't join the team. He was a horrible coach, so I trained mostly on my own. I never played basketball on the school team. I had to work in the afternoons, so going to basketball practices would have lost me money. I had bought a real home. I couldn't afford to not work full-time while I went to high school and had a mortgage to pay. I was fourteen years old with too much responsibility on my shoulders.

But I could run anytime. Running was my escape from a violent household, from a family that couldn't make enough money to keep the electricity on, from not knowing how to act like a teenager. Even when I got drunk with friends in high school (I fell in with the wrong crowd, looking for acceptance), I would go running around the park after a few beers at night as my "friends" continued to drink sitting on a park table. I felt free and in control of who and what I was when I ran. I tried to run between one hundred to one hundred twenty miles a week as a fourteen- and fifteen-year-old.

Races were few and far between back then, and I entered some half-marathons in 1980 and the beginning of 1981. I entered my first marathon down in the Los Angeles area. (I thought it was called the Santa Monica Marathon, but I haven't been able to find it since then, and nothing like it exists anymore.) My mom and I planned to start the three-hour car drive to the race at 3:00 a.m. My mother surprised me with a new turquoise singlet and matching shorts to wear for the race. I had never had matching running clothes; this was a very special gift. (If you know me now, you know I take great pride in my matching work clothes and racing clothes. I always feel that if I dress up, I will do better. I blame my mom for this clothing and shoe fetish.)

I was shocked when I got up in the morning to find my father dressed and ready to go. He had even warmed up the car. He drove us to the race while I slept in the back seat. When we arrived, my father's embarrassment at not feeling like he fit in was so apparent. This was a new world for him: skinny people in tiny shorts and singlets. He had never exercised a day in his life. After he parked the car, I got my number at the registration desk and said goodbye to my parents as I went to the lineup at the starting line. Signs were posted in the starting shoot for minutes per mile (9:00 min., 8:30, 8:00, etc.). I was shooting for an 8:15-minute-per-mile pace for the marathon, so I lined up quietly to the side of the timing sign.

I watched men warming up, running up and down the sidewalks, skipping, stretching, doing (what seemed to me at the time) bizarre things. I couldn't even imagine why they were wasting their energy before running 26.2 miles. There were very few women lining up for the race; I spotted maybe three. I waited patiently, watching everything, and then I just ran with everyone when the gun went off. I was completely overwhelmed and scared.

I don't remember the beginning of the race at all. I just kept going. I don't remember reading the mile markers, though I know I must have seen some. At mile twenty, I lost it mentally. Completely. Back then, people on the sidelines told you where you were if you were a front racer; we didn't have GPS watches. After a water station, I was physically and mentally struggling, and a man got in my face and yelled, "Sixth!" I can still picture his face.

I stopped dead, completely bewildered, and was looking backward toward the water station I had just passed. There was no way we were only at mile six! I couldn't do it. I started crying and wanted to give up. Then, an older man in his sixties said, "Oh no, you are the sixth woman. See that woman up there ahead of us? She is number five. You can catch her." I was delirious and couldn't comprehend what he was saying as he pointed ahead to a group of runners.

"Here, just run with me. I will stay with you," he said. And I did. I ran hard, cried, stayed with him, and ran like I did almost two years earlier on that first morning when I ran my first twenty-three steps. I came around a corner and saw the finish line with the flags flapping in the wind. My father leaned against a power pole with his back to me, smoking a cigarette. I knew him from his cheap western boots and his too-short pants. My mother saw me and started yelling, "There she is! There she is!" beating her fists on my father's arm. Spectators screamed and clapped on the street as the runners headed toward the finish line. My father turned around and looked at me in complete shock with his mouth hanging open, his cigarette dangling from his hand by his leg. I ran as fast as I could for that finish line and passed out cold as soon as I crossed it.

I came to the medic tent with an IV in me and a blood pressure cuff on. I was chafing, bleeding, hurting all over, cramping, and dizzy. None of that mattered, though. I was deliriously happy. I smiled so much my cheeks hurt. My mother stood outside the medic tent, looking very worried about the state I was in. She had never seen a human being sick from too much exercise. "Mom, can you find the man that helped me finish? A man ran with me the last six miles and helped me to the finish. I need to thank him." That was my concern, to thank the man that helped me run and finish the marathon. I had run and finished a full marathon! I was now a marathoner with a shirt and everything!

"Vanessa, you were running alone when you came around the corner? What man are you talking about?"

I felt lost and sad. I so wanted to thank the man that helped me finish my first marathon. I will never know if the man was real or just a hallucination. I still think he was real. I look for him at every race I go to now forty years later even though I know he must have passed away by now. But what mattered most was I was the first female in the under-eighteen division of a marathon—a full flipping 26.2-mile marathon!

I slept for three days after that marathon and couldn't walk for a week. I was so happy and proud of myself for what I accomplished, I couldn't stop smiling. This was a different kind of happiness and pride; it was internal. In 1982, I ran two more marathons, with one being close to my hometown in Nipomo, CA, called the Joker's Wild 5 Mile and Marathon.

Want to know the best part? I won that one as the first overall female. I still have the shirt after all these years, and it now hangs in the bathroom of my fitness studio in San Jose, CA. I touch it every day to remember how running has changed my life.

I tore my Achilles tendon in my senior year of high school. Those one-hundred-twenty-mile weeks caught up with me without proper training and coaching. But in the 1980s, we just didn't know better as runners. We just ran.

Your body is a gift that can bring you great joy no matter what you are doing with it. I treat my body well to avoid injury and take care of it in sports and generally in life now. I have found that when I can make my body perform well, I am also mentally happier.

This is the message I want to pass on in this health and fitness book, a happier you physically and mentally.

So, let's get started.

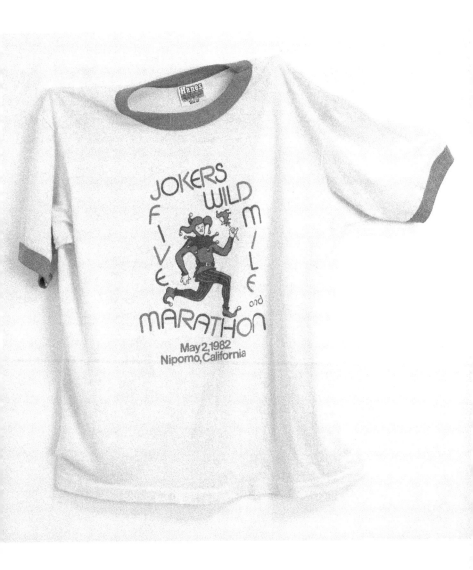

# PART 2

# LIVING IN YOUR BODY

# CHAPTER 4

# MY PERSONAL PAIN

We all have different reasons to want to be fit and healthy. For all the reasons clients have ever come to me, or friends or acquaintances have ever asked me questions about their bodies, the common factor is *pain*. Mental and physical pain.

As a child, I was in constant pain. I was fat and unable to move my body in the ways I wanted, and I was sad and depressed about this all the time. I didn't have any friends. The only solution I knew was drowning my sorrows in sugar. I consumed my jealousy and rage. It was everyone else's fault I was fat and unattractive. My parents were poor and un-athletic, my father beat me, my siblings were drug addicts, and no one tried to help me. There were no real role models in my life for health and happiness, except Father Colberg. He was my parish priest in grade school.

Santa Maria was a small town when I was young, and everyone had horses. My parents didn't have much money so they bought me the cheapest horse they could find, Phantom. She was a crazy bay mare that came with a saddle, brushes, bridle, halter—everything you needed to own a horse. The asking price was two hundred and fifty dollars. We got her with everything for one hundred and fifty dollars. Phantom tried to kill me every day. She would buck me off and pin me in her stall, smashing me against a wall. I tried to tame that crazy mare. At the local stable where I boarded her and worked cleaning stalls, there were horse shows once a month on the first Saturday of the month. These stables were directly across from the mobile home park where we lived.

On Horse Show Day, my father would drink beer with the other dads, and the young girls would show their pretty horses in their pretty matching show clothes. My horse Phantom and I would just cause chaos. She would buck me off, run around the arena into the other calm horses and riders. I would wear the wrong outfit and just look foolish. I never placed in the horse show classes except last. Every show, I would end up crying for hours afterward from shame and embarrassment. After another disastrous Saturday Horse Show, my drunken father told me my problem was that I didn't pray to God and go to church enough. All I needed to do was pray a Novena for thirty days, and then I would do great at my next horse show.

So, to the great calls of laughter from my grade school class-mates after school, I would go to the Catholic Church across the playground when school got out to pray the Stations of the Cross. I put up with the mental pain of being embarrassed in front of my schoolmates for going to church because I thought I would get a reward at the end of the month. I was going to do great at my horse show because God would appreciate all these prayers! I did this praying every day after school for an entire month. It was just the old ladies with their boobs hanging down to their waists and ugly big-heeled black shoes and I in the church every afternoon. This Novena took about an hour every day.

The Saturday Horse Show came around. I got dressed up in the clothes sewn by my father because we couldn't afford store-bought show clothes. I tried to show my horse and poof—she stepped on my foot, got loose, and ran around like crazy, run-ning into other horses and people just as she had done the month before. Even my dad laughed this time so hard he fell on a wire and cut his leg. He had to go to the hospital to get stitches.

I was humiliated again and in mental pain from my horse per-forming poorly. I now knew I was fat and looked stupid in my cheap-looking horse show clothes. My drunken father's behav-ior didn't help. Add this with the physical pain of my horse step-ping on my foot. Obviously, there was no God present then to help me. Why did God allow me to have this much pain when I had spent so much time praying to Him?

I steamed and steamed in my thoughts over this fiasco that was supposed to be my winning horse show. I had decided to give up crying. Crying obviously didn't help. Crying helped about as much as the praying did. I stayed in bed all day on Sunday and let rage fester. I read books and ate candy. Candy and large amounts of sugar had always been my comfort as a child.

I went to school on Monday and didn't talk to anyone all day. After school, I walked over to the church, seeing the same six ladies wasting their time praying. I grabbed the hymnals out from the back of the pews and threw them hard at the altar, screaming at God, "You are fake, and you don't exist! I hate you!" A woman younger than most of the women in the church (mid-forties, dignified looking, thin, well dressed) came over to me and whispered, "Leave this church immediately. You are causing a disturbance." Her whisper came out like a hiss.

"Shut up, and leave me alone. I have a right to be here and do whatever I want. You are a drunk just like my father!" I screamed at her, and immediately she slapped me, hard, right across my face. This stranger had hit an obviously poor, out-of-control fat child. I was eleven years old.

"Oh no, no, no," said Father Colberg as he hurried into the church with his long black robes flowing behind him. He told the woman to leave the church immediately. Father Colberg took my hand and helped me pick up the hymnals I had thrown at the altar. He was reticent. He sat me down in a pew, then turned to me and asked, "Vanessa, why are you so angry at God?"

"Father, I came to this church every day after school and prayed a Novena for a whole month so that I would do better at my horse show. It didn't work. I still did horrible, and everyone laughed at me." My nose was bleeding from the slap of the woman, and I cried this blood and snot all over the cassock of Father Colberg.

Father Colberg took out a folded handkerchief from his pocket and handed it to me. He looked at me with the kindest eyes ever and said, "Vanessa, what the hell were you doing in this church praying every day after school for an hour instead of working with that damn horse? How is that horse going to get better with you here? Don't you know that doing the best you can do, with everything God has given you, your body, and your mind, is the best prayer to God you can ever do? I watch you, Vanessa. I notice that you never apply yourself at anything. Not with your schoolwork, not with your appearance, not with making friends, not with anything. I never want to see you wasting your time in this church praying again. Vanessa, you study, get good grades, and work that horse to the best of your ability, and God will reward you. God rewards people who work hard."

That afternoon was such a turning point in my life. I went home and thought about Father Colberg's speech and the slap of that woman for weeks. I looked around at my parents, my siblings, my classmates, and people on television, and I thought, *Did they have good lives because of good luck, or did they work hard for the things they wanted?* No one in my life worked hard at anything, really. I had a family of complainers and blamers. My father couldn't keep a job for more than three months because he always thought he was smarter than the boss. My father was constantly getting fired.

I was tired of being in physical and mental pain. I didn't know how to fix most of the pain, but I had to start somewhere. I fixed my grades first and became a good student. I tried to be polite to everyone, even if I was jealous or they were mean to me. I stopped blaming others when I failed at school, or with my horse, or at anything and questioned myself. Had I put in the work to succeed? And if I hadn't put in a serious effort, I asked myself how I put in the work next time to succeed to avoid anger and disappointment. I stopped being jealous of other families' money and good looks and, instead, concentrated on the parts of me that I could control and change.

I have lived a far from perfect life, but I always take the time to evaluate when things aren't going the way I want them to and figure out what I, and not everyone else, am doing wrong and how I can change.

I don't ignore pain anymore. I study the pain I am in—*Is it physical, mental, or both, and where did this pain come from?* This constant evaluation has helped me accept and better myself.

# CHAPTER 5

# EVALUATING YOUR OWN PAIN

L et's analyze your pain so we can move forward with a plan for your body. Pain is not weakness. We all have pain in our bodies, and we need to recognize what kind of pain it is, so we can properly address it.

Privately, answer these questions about your pain:

1.  Is my pain emotional or physical? Sometimes my pain is physical and brought on by my actions. I drank too much alcohol or sugary drinks, overate, didn't exercise, or overslept. Did these activities hurt my body enough to cause depression? Are they the reason I am not able to show up fully for work or other day-to-day

activities? Am I carrying extra weight that is hurting my joints? I need to analyze what my pain is, so I can move forward.

2. If my pain is physical, do I need to see a doctor? Have I been putting off physicals because I am too scared to know what is wrong? Am I eating, drinking, sleeping, and exercising well? In other words, is my physical pain self-inflected? Such a tough question. I know seeing a doctor is difficult and expensive in our current climate, but it's better to know and get simple things checked. I suggest a blood test annually to all my clients so they can monitor their health properly. Check your blood pressure regularly. Blood pressure cuffs are cheap, and every house should have one.

3. Did I cause this pain? If I physically caused my body to hurt, then how is my mind coping with that? Am I anxious, depressed, obsessive, angry, and jealous? Is that mental pain causing my life to be worse? Am I taking the pain out on myself or those around me?

I have worked with many clients from all aspects of life, and pain is a common thread with *everyone*. You are not alone. When you are a personal trainer and spend two to three hours a week with a client one-on-one, you get to know all of your clients well, and every one of them has shared their pain with me as we try to move on to a better place in their lives.

I am now going to describe some pain issues I have seen in my clients. You will hear more in upcoming chapters. I want you to realize other people experience the same pain.

## THE PAIN OF BEING OVERWEIGHT/OBESE

In the United States, we have an obesity rate of over forty percent and an overweight population of over thirty-five percent. This means that only twenty-five percent of Americans are at a "healthy weight."

The pain of being overweight has many manifestations, from being unable to move comfortably, being tired all the time, and having knee, back, and ankle pain. Obese people also have diseases caused by this excess weight, such as diabetes, heart problems, circulation problems, etc. But these are the common problems everyone recognizes from being overweight. Let's talk about some real reasons why my overweight clients came to see me.

They can't wipe their own butts when they go to the bathroom because they can't reach their arms around their large bodies to their backsides. With their current weight, they are unable to clean themselves after urination or defecation. This problem occurs with many clients who need to lose sixty pounds or more. Obese and overweight people consume so much food in a day that they go to the bathroom many times in twenty-four hours. Paid caretakers or loved ones help them with all day-to-day activities. Due to their poor hygiene, they get bacterial infections often and have gastrointestinal problems constantly. Burping and farting uncontrollably is common. The obese/overweight person just ignores this passing of gas, as do their family members, to try to control the embarrassment.

Many obese people can't dress themselves. Obese women can't put on and latch their own bras, so they stop wearing them, and the weight of their breasts causes more back pain. They call their husbands or children in to help them dress, causing more humiliation.

If a person is more than eighty pounds overweight, their legs usually look red. The skin is overly tight and stretched, and the pores began to ooze pus. Special medical wraps have been developed for this medical condition. These wraps cause compression on the lower leg and keep bacteria from developing in the open wounds. The leg wraps need to be changed, cleaned, and dried daily by someone one else because the obese person cannot bend over and take care of this condition themselves.

Furniture often breaks beneath obese people. Chairs break, if they can fit in them. Tables and counters break from being leaned on. Obese people who need to lose sixty pounds or more are so large that the extra weight creates pressure on their lungs, so they cannot breathe. To sleep, they need to be propped up in a bed or, more commonly, use a recliner to sleep. Sleep apnea is common because the human body wakes up when it can't get enough oxygen during sleep. This causes a cycle of insufficient sleep which also increases cravings for sugary and carbohydrate-laden foods.

Due to the exertion of just trying to do daily activities, obese people are hot and sweat most of the time with small movements. Anxiety is common over this sweating problem. Obese and overweight people commonly feel like they are overheating. They keep their homes very cold to avoid overheating and sweating, which causes rashes. Overweight people use talcum powder in the creases of their skin to sooth their sores. They are also embarrassed in public about their excessive sweating; they wipe their foreheads and necks with towels or napkins. Working out is embarrassing because they sweat so much; they often apologize for it. This overheating also makes it difficult to work out, raising their heart rates and blood pressure to dangerous and painful levels.

When a human being is overweight, their bellies stick out in front of their bodies, causing their backs to arch to hold everything up and counterbalance their weight. This back arch causes back pain and knee pain. The pressure on their lungs from this belly fat keeps them from taking full breathes when they bend over. Unfortunately, overweight men can no longer look down and see their penises for urination, or cleaning, or having sex. I have worked with many men who are one hundred pounds overweight, and their humiliation that they can no longer be sexual is heartbreaking.

Overweight women develop yeast infections and bacterial urinary tract infections due to the excess fat that grows around their vaginas, which causes pain and discomfort.

Most obese people don't have sex anymore, which causes them to feel unimportant to their spouses or feel very sexually unattractive. As a result, they cut off the sexual part of their lives.

I will talk about food and dietary needs in a later chapter at length and many times when I discuss my actual clients, but let's talk about eating in general with overweight individuals. Most overweight people eat in private to avoid being judged for their food intake. They have become good at lying to themselves about what and how much they eat. Food delivery is the number-one tool used by overweight people to get food. It can be Safeway, Target, DoorDash, Uber Eats, or any pizza delivery restaurant. By getting their food delivered, they can buy food without many people looking at them and judging them. Going to the grocery store can be humiliating, but with delivery, only one person sees you: the driver. Once, a woman, with potato chip crumbs around her mouth, looked me in the eye and told me she couldn't understand how she could be so overweight when all she ate was vegetables. These crumbs extended to her computer, where she sat all day playing video games. Yes, technically, potatoes are vegetables, but she knew better. I never confront a client in that moment because they know they are lying to themselves, and to me. They need to get through the lies themselves first.

*Confrontation never works when you are trying to help*
*people. Confrontation creates anger and resentment.*

Obese people can be defiant about their food consumption. I had a woman consume over twelve thousand calories one evening because *she wanted to*. She didn't care about her commitment she had made previously. She liked food and felt like eating it. It made her feel better. She had consumed so much food the day before that exercise was impossible. She was sick from overeating. I will discuss this woman at great length later in the book. This is a very important story.

I watched a three-hundred-fifty-pound woman pull her car up to a burger joint. The car was tilted to the driver's side by her weight. She had to do this rocking motion to get out of the car and catch her breath. Then, she walked into the burger place. She bought six hamburgers and, huffing just from the walk back to her car, fell back into her car. With her legs still hanging out of the open door, she ate each burger as quickly as she could in two to three bites. Her arms and neck were full of rashes. I was just leaving my fitness studio and said, "I'm going for a jog. Throw those remaining burgers away, and I will give you a free workout."

She looked at me and laughed, "No, eating all these burgers is more fun. F— you." She then threw her burger wrappers at me. I saw the pain in her eyes and knew she was lashing out. I picked up her trash and just went on my run.

## CROOKED BODIES, HURTING FROM AGE, ACCIDENTS, OR LACK OF USE

Look at professional athletes. Their bodies are straight from the top of their heads to their ankles and straight across their shoulders. Many people walk into my studio with their necks three to five inches in front of their chests and their heads permanently looking down to the ground in front of them. Some have one shoulder higher than the other, a hip that doesn't work and won't rotate; back pain, foot pain, and knee pain are all common ailments. Many people have modified their lives to fit their aches and pains instead of fixing the muscular parts of their bodies to get out of pain. Making people's posture straight is a priority for me. All of my workouts are about good posture and understanding how your body is supposed to work.

### AGING AND IN CONSTANT PAIN

I get many clients who are sixty-five years old and older who can barely walk or get out of a chair by using only their legs and not pushing off their arms. They have never been physically active and are realizing the damage this has done to their bodies. Even if they aren't drastically overweight, just getting out of bed and walking around the block is uncomfortable and painful. In fact, walking can be scary because they may fall down and cause a serious injury.

Because of this lack of physical work in their lives, they have no muscle development, causing their skeletal system to break down. I had a client who was proud to call herself an "energy conserver" her entire life. She could barely walk when I met her seven years ago, but now, she walks two miles every day while listening to podcasts. She realizes how much better she feels when she moves. Just FYI, that didn't happen overnight. This change for the better took *years.*

## SO MANY PRESCRIPTION MEDICATIONS

Our medical professionals have become pill pushers. There is no other way to say it. People go to the doctor not feeling well and expect to walk out of the doctor's office with a prescription for a pill to fix them. Many doctors have told me their patients don't want to hear that a poor diet and lack of exercise have caused their medical issues. Doctors prescribe them diabetes medications, heart medications, blood pressure medications, anxiety pills, etc. Doctors rarely broach lifestyle changes.

All of these medications damage kidneys, the liver, bladder, etc. When people take lots of medicines that interact adversely, they feel worse. This causes them more mental and physical pain. Doctors also hate to take clients off medications because once you have gone on the medication and the client feels better, taking them off could get them sick again. This is a bad circular situation.

## PLASTIC SURGERY WON'T HEAL MENTAL PAIN

I believe we should all get to dress or do whatever we want to with our bodies because it is our choice. I don't have a problem with tattoos or piercings, thirteen different shades of colored hair, wearing a burka, or whatever. But if you are doing extreme things because you are trying to stop the aging process and those injections or operations have damaged your body, well then, we now have a problem. A woman walked into my studio with her breasts so large that they were coming out of the sides of her bra by her arms. When she moved the left arm over her head, the breast implant moved up under her chin. She could never get the sculpted arms she wanted because she had damaged the pectoral muscle that extended from the chest to her arm; she couldn't run or jump without extreme pain. She wore two bras all the time.

Having liposuction is an extreme surgery done with a large needle inserted and suction down, pulling out the fat cells in your abdomen, legs, butt, or other areas. The fat continues oozing out over a couple of weeks. Watch this on YouTube and see how violent this surgery is to the human body. You can do this with diet and exercise. Resorting to surgery is the easy way out but very painful and expensive. Besides, the scars are apparent to anyone who sees you without clothes.

Women have come to me after these plastic surgeries, not happy with the results. The fat came back, or their breasts look wrong, and still, they know they aren't healthy and need to work out to get the physical body they desire.

## ANOREXIA, EATING DISORDERS, FOOD ALLERGIES, AND OTHER REASONS PEOPLE DON'T EAT

Before I became a personal trainer, I never saw the damage of anorexia and bulimia. Sure, I saw overweight people and people who looked overly thin but never up close and personal. When people don't eat enough calories or nutrients, they are exhausted and irritable, sleeping twelve to eighteen hours a day to cope. Working, having a relationship, and fulfilling day-to-day activities seem impossible under these conditions. Depression and mood swings frequently arise due to the lack of nutrition and exercise. Stomach acid and other stomach issues make them feel sick when they work out, so they continue to not move their bodies. Joints and bones break down from the lack of nutrients. Stress fractures and other injuries are common.

I hope you could recognize yourself or your loved ones in the above examples. Pain is real, even when self-inflicted, and it needs to be acknowledged and cared for, not judged.

# CHAPTER 6

# HONESTY IS HARD.
# BEING HUMAN IS HARD.

*I* want you to read this chapter alone, so you can be perfectly honest with yourself and not worry about being judged by others or even judging yourself. Find some paper and write down your thoughts, not necessarily your answers.

Thoughts, feelings, and answers are not the same. Remember, this is just you reading to understand yourself, so don't be concerned about (even your own) judgment.

Ask yourself these questions:

1. Do I physically hurt when I get up in the morning? Is it a struggle to get out of bed? Do I have to use my arms

and crawl to get up and get my feet on the floor? Do my shoulders and hips hurt after sleeping on my side? How old is my bed? (We spend a third of our lives in our beds, and oftentimes, they are worn out and hurt us. Buy a new mattress every five to six years.) Do I worry about hurting myself just getting out of bed? Have I actually hurt myself in my sleep or getting out of bed like a crooked neck or back pain or leg pain? Why can't I get out of bed easily?

2. Have I ever broken a table, chair, toilet, or sink from leaning on it to get up or move around? Can I get up on my legs from a chair or sofa without using my arms to push off?

3. Can I do everyday tasks like jump up to get something off a shelf, twist open a jar of pickles, or chase after the mailman—because I forgot to leave a letter to be mailed successfully—and not feel foolish, fall down, or hurt myself?

4. Can I fit into my clothes comfortably without being out of breath and blaming the dryer for shrinking my jeans again?

5. Do I like the way I look in a mirror? (This question is difficult to answer. Stand there naked and look at yourself. Don't judge what is "wrong"; marvel at the human body and what can be done with it.)

6. Am I embarrassed about my protruding stomach, flabby arms, second chin, etc.? Do I choose clothes that hide my body? (If you are a woman and you use Spanx...just stop! There is no way putting your body in a piece of elastic is right for your internal organs.)

7. Do I feel I am attractive, physically and emotionally—not just sexually to someone but generally to other people?

8. What physical things have I always wanted to do—run a marathon, snow or water ski, hike a mountain, bench two hundred pounds, travel to Europe or Africa, or pick up and hold my grandchildren? Why haven't I been able to do these things? Have I been even too scared to try to do things physically for fear of failure or hurting myself?

9. How often have I vowed to start a diet and exercise program "tomorrow" and never started? How often have I spent money on a gym membership, workout DVDs, or exercise equipment that has gone unused? Why do I spend the money and then never start exercising even when I want to and know exercise is good for me?

10. Do I criticize runners ("Runners are always injuring themselves, and people die in marathons all the time!"), men with six-pack abs and great arms ("They are just gym obsessed and self-centered!"), women with great

legs and flat stomachs ("Must be plastic surgery!"), and athletic-looking people ("Oh, they were probably born that way.") when deep down I'm jealous? Am I unwilling to put in the work to look or feel like them? Does this criticism of them make me feel better?

*And the big one...*

11. Why don't I look and feel the way I want to?

Lying is a coping mechanism. We lie to avoid the pain of the truth. Sometimes the truth just sucks. Being honest with yourself helps you grow spiritually and physically.

So, here's how to start being honest with yourself about your body:

*Write it down.*

Grab some blank pieces of paper, and on the top, write the days and dates for one week. All goals need to be obtainable. Vow only to yourself that you will write about your body every day for two minutes at the end of every day. Just two minutes.

Example: *Monday, June 2, 2020—I did not exercise. I ate three Big Macs. I drank beer and no water. I meditated for three minutes.*

That is more than enough! This is not a *Write down your goals* exercise; this is a *Can I be honest with myself?* daily exercise.

At the end of seven days, go back and read through your week and make adjustments to know you weren't completely honest with yourself. For example, it wasn't three Big Macs; it was four. Don't get mad for lying to yourself. Just fix it and move forward, trying to be as honest as possible the first time through.

Being honest with ourselves gives us a starting point. Now let's learn about our bodies and how we can work with them to make ourselves feel better physically and emotionally.

# CHAPTER 7

# UNDERSTAND WHAT YOUR BODY NEEDS

This isn't a book with a quick description of a diet and exercise program. No, this is a book that will hopefully take you on a lifelong journey to better health and loving the body you live in. Embark on a journey of discovering what you currently have, what you want, what you need to get there, and how to get there. First, let's review your body and how you relate to it.

When I work with a client, I try not to give them a diet, an exercise, or any mental work that I don't think they can accomplish. Failure is not an option. Failing, even on a small new endeavor, makes us doubt ourselves. My job as a personal trainer is to try to help people have the bodies that allow them to enjoy life and create a desire for improvement and accomplishment with their bodies and minds. Please take this same mindset as you try to move forward. Be gentle with yourself and take small steps toward big improvements over time. Realize this body transformation will take time.

If I start with a fifty-eight-year-old woman who has never worked out, I don't expect her to go out and run five miles and curl fifteen-pound dumbbells on the first try. I am realistic and supportive.

I am famous for asking my clients, "Have I ever given a count you couldn't do?" Not one client has ever been able to answer, "Yes, yesterday!"

When you first buy a car, a puppy, or even those five-hundred-dollar fancy boots, you strive to take care of those new objects that are important and precious to you. You want to enjoy these things for a long time. You wash and wax that new car every week. You feed, water, and cuddle the dog. And you don't ever go in the rain with those hot new boots that you still keep in the original box. (Here is a personal disclosure: I was on a bad date, having dinner about a mile from my hotel. The date was so bad I wanted to sneak out the back of the restaurant and leave. Problem? I was wearing thousand-dollar high-heeled Italian red boots that I absolutely loved and took me three months to pay off. Solution? Ask the kitchen staff for plastic bags to cover my feet and carry the boots, so I could jog back to my hotel room and save my boots from possible damage. Conclusion? I chose damaging my ego over damaging those boots. I looked like a fool jogging down a major street in a big city with plastic bags on my feet, slapping my feet on the concrete and laughing the whole way back to my hotel. It was actually kind of fun.)

So, why don't we feel the same about our physical bodies? Why do we do things to our bodies that cause short- and long-term pain, when we wouldn't do so to a prized possession like the boots I just discussed?

The first concept for the new you: you have control over your body. You control what you put into it, as in food, drugs, liquids, creams, and/or alcohol. You also have control over what you do physically with your body: Sit on the couch and watch television for six hours. Play video games for eight hours at a stretch. Sleep too little or all day. Exercise. Hit yourself with a hammer. Walk the dog. Have sex with six strangers in a day. Whatever you do, you have to understand that what we do physically to our body affects us mentally also.

All of us have done things—ate a whole box of See's Candy in one sitting, drank four margaritas in an hour, stayed up too late watching television—that affected our activities for the next few days. If we took twenty-three seconds to think about that activity before we did it, actually counting those seconds out to give us pause, would we still do that activity? Now twenty-three happens to be my favorite number, and just long enough for me to think about the ramifications of my actions but not long enough to create havoc, so it works for me. (Also, twenty-three is the first number of steps I ever ran and why I named my company Fitness 23.) Pick a number that works for you but make it at least a count to ten. Make a promise to yourself to think about your body and if the action you are about to take will get you where you want to be in the future.

We only get this one body, and our bodies are far from perfect. No one has a perfect body. Every professional athlete works hard at his or her craft and fitness to excel in their chosen sport. Just having significant genes doesn't win your tennis tournaments or help you run marathons. If pretty people eat junk food and drink beer all day, they aren't physically or mentally attractive anymore either.

We all have these different bodies that, with work and care, can be better. Let's learn how.

We don't have to be doctors to take care of these amazing machines, but let's start with a few simple concepts.

We humans are in a symbiotic and intertwined relationship with these needs: water, shelter, sleep, food, and exercise. Plain and simple. We need to meet all five of these with as little physical and mental stress in our daily lives. When one aspect of this relationship fails, the whole ship starts to tilt. Then the sinking begins.

*WATER*

The first concept to grasp is our need for water. Our bodies are sixty to seventy percent water. Dehydration causes many health issues such as rapid heartbeat, dizziness, sleeplessness, headaches, and fainting. The first step to improving your health is consistently drinking enough water. Never allow yourself to be dehydrated, especially before going to sleep. Going to sleep dehydrated makes you wake up with a headache—a rough start to a new day.

My standard starting point for all clients is thirty ounces of water first thing in the morning before your coffee or tea and thirty ounces of water again around 2:00 or 3:00 p.m. This amount of water is drunk all at once, in a minute or less. The time of day can change slightly, but the amount of water consumed needs to be at least thirty ounces. It is typical for me to drink close to fifty ounces of water in the afternoons between 3:00 and 7:00 p.m. My body just tells me it needs water from the eight miles I ran in the morning, the nine clients I worked out with, and is getting ready for the next day. I listen to my body carefully. The afternoon time for drinking water needs to fit your schedule. So you are close to a bathroom. Don't drink so much water too late in the evening, or the urge to urinate could ruin your sleep. When you first start drinking lots of water, you may feel like you are urinating constantly. On the flip side, your body may also hold this water and make you feel bloated for the first few days. Don't worry. As your body gets used to your new daily water intake, it will adjust.

Not drinking plain water causes gastrointestinal problems along with kidney pain, bladder conditions, and skin problems. If a client tells me, "I just can't drink water; I hate it," I try anything to get them to try drinking at least a small amount of water. We do smaller amounts, even just sips, and work up to thirty ounces. Don't make this water drinking a punishment. We can add cucumbers, berries, or lemon to the water to change the taste or even add a powdered electrolyte mix if completely necessary—anything to just get water in our system. Be adjustable. Don't expect this to be easy. This is a tough, significant life change.

I have a new client. She is a beautiful tech worker in her late twenties. She came to me to lose about thirty pounds and kickstart an exercise program. I just see her one day a week. After three weeks, she walked into the studio, positively glowing! I smiled, and she said, "Wow, just look at my skin. It looks beautiful!" She hadn't lost any weight yet, common for the first three weeks. (The body holds on to the weight, but I will discuss this in upcoming chapters.) However, her water consumption had flushed toxins from her skin. What a great starting point on her fitness journey! We all need small rewards.

### SHELTER

We all live in the nicest houses we can afford, but that is not all I am referring to with shelter. I'm talking about fulfilling basic needs, asking yourself questions like, *Am I too cold or too hot? Do I dress comfortably in the day? Does my work environment make me feel comfortable, physically and mentally?* If these needs are not met the body will be under stress. Stress is a killer. Poor office air conditioners, uncomfortable office chairs, improper computer angles—all need to be addressed. Living in noisy, cluttered homes can also be upsetting. Figure out what living conditions make you happiest mentally and work toward that ideal.

### SLEEP

First, you spend one-third of your life in bed, so invest in a great mattress and bedding that makes you feel great when you wake up. Plan to buy a new mattress every five to six years. I sleep with my dogs every night, so it's hard to sleep without them when I travel. Sleeping with pets would gross many people out, so do what works for you. I also need to make my bed every morning because I like to sleep in a clean, tidy bed.

Understand your sleep comfort needs and your own personal sleep cycle for optimum health. Pick two days in a row that you don't need to be anywhere at specific morning times. When you start to feel tired, shut off all electronics and make sure that all lights, including lights from chargers, are not in your eyesight. Read an actual book if you need help falling asleep. I use a fitness watch to monitor my sleep. Most tech watches can track and monitor sleep and oxygen levels now, so you can learn how much deep, light, and REM sleep you get daily and need to thrive. Wake up without an alarm and see how you feel. If you still feel exhausted, it could be you don't get at least two to three hours of deep sleep. Now analyze why you did or didn't wake up feeling refreshed. Did you eat at least three hours before going to bed? How was your alcohol intake? Sugar intake? Did you eat a large dinner with meat before bed? Try to monitor these as it relates to your sleep patterns. Be honest with yourself and try minor modifications to see if they can help your sleep. Everyone is different. I can eat dinner and then fall asleep in twenty minutes, but many people can't.

Because of our life needs, kids, and jobs, we can't always dictate when we wake up. I am an early riser, and my body prefers to get up at 4:30 a.m. I run early in the morning and do my office work afterward, and I feel very productive spending my early morning time this way. I go to sleep around 8:00 to 9:00 p.m. Figure out what works best for you to get that deep solid sleep and a minimum of seven hours total sleep every day. I am very physically active in the day, so two or three days a week, I also nap for thirty minutes or so. Sleep is so essential for daily function, and as we add movement and dietary changes, we want all these regular phases of our lives to help each other, not hinder each other.

Now for the toughest part of our relationship with our body: food.

## THE STARTING POINT: HONESTY AND SOME SELF-DISCOVERY

What do you eat on a daily basis? Make an actual food journal of everything you put in your mouth for at least seven days straight. Include additives like creamer, sugar, salt, salsa, etc.

How many times a day do you eat, and where do you eat? Make sure to include all times. For example, *an apple at 10:00 a.m. in my car* would be an extra mealtime. *A handful of pistachios at my desk around 3:00 p.m.*—oh, was it a handful or a bag?

Are you eating for pleasure, to occupy your hands, or from boredom? Don't forget to add this to your food journal. We need to understand why you are eating.

Do you ever feel hungry? What does hunger feel like? Describe it.

Do you just eat because it is time? It's noon—shouldn't I eat some lunch?

When you eat, do you feel nauseous afterward? Do you know why you feel sick after you eat?

Do you eat very fast? Are you scared someone will catch you or take your food away? Why do you eat so fast? Do you get pleasure from eating quickly?

Do you snack many times a day? Do you realize how many times a day you eat outside of your normal mealtimes? Jot this down in your food journal.

Do you hide food in places that aren't the kitchen, like your car, office desk, or nightstand? Remember, no one needs to see these answers. This is just for you to understand your relationship with food and have a conversation with yourself about it.

Have you ever been disgusted with yourself after you ate?

Do you make promises to yourself—"I will stop eating sugar!"—then break that promise almost immediately?

Let's start a new relationship and conversation with food so the food we consume can help us to make our bodies feel energetic and content. Eating food should make us feel good, not bad. Don't try to change everything at once when it comes to your food choices. The first step is to understand that your body is a machine; it needs to be fueled just like your car. The farther you drive, the more gas and oil it needs. I plan my food, water, and sleep about twelve hours before I begin my daily activities.

Here's an example: I am going on a six-mile run tomorrow morning. I have to consume over sixty ounces of water in the afternoon before my run, or I will be dehydrated when I wake up in the morning. By 6:00 p.m., I will eat a dinner that is light on my stomach—no red meat, as it takes too long to digest, and no heavy dairy, which upsets my stomach. I finish dinner, giving myself a good three hours to digest, so I can get to sleep by 9:00 p.m. I sleep until 4:30 am. I am over fifty, and gosh, I miss great sleep. I try for eight hours of sleep every night but can function well on seven hours. If I can stick to my routine, I will wake up with no stomach issues, go to the bathroom, drink half a cup of coffee, and go out to have a successful run and start my day.

After looking at your food journal, you can see how you currently eat in a week. Let's talk about it. Do you eat food at home, or do you eat out often? Are you eating alone or with others? Are you able to classify your food? Protein, vegetables, fruits, carbohydrates, and drinks are the only classifications that matter to me initially. A secondary look will start to separate processed foods.

When I get a food journal from a client, I ask them what they believe is important to do on a daily basis. Do they have dinner with their family every evening? If so, we definitely keep that meal. We are humans who have other humans around us. Do you exercise in the morning, do you drink alcohol in the evenings? Is wine important to you? If you enjoy alcohol (I sure do! I used to be a sommelier), then keep the alcohol in but just be cognizant that it contains sugar, which can disrupt your sleep, so try to drink moderately. Avoid mixed drinks that are adding more sugar with concentrated juices. For example, instead of a margarita, it could be tequila over ice with a splash of lime juice. Simple modifications.

I never want to completely change someone's daily eating habits. The idea is to be successful in small steps. The first step I take with a client is taking out as much processed food as possible. Have them understand what processed food is. Our American diet and grocery stores are full of processed food, and this is, in my opinion, the reason we are so fat as a society. We eat processed food with very little nutritional value. Because our bodies aren't getting the nutrition they need and are asking for, we eat even more food, and cravings happen.

If it comes in a bag or box and contains more than three items, it is processed food. Now, I avoid processed food as much as possible. I make exceptions for some things in my own diet, but I buy these items fresh to avoid preservatives. I purchase bagels and bread from bakeries or the farmer's market. These have minimal ingredients, less than ten, and no preservatives. I still eat food prepared by others (just not by large production companies) ninety percent of the time. I was an organic farmer in my previous career, so I always buy organic when I can. Learning to enjoy cooking will broaden your food choices.

I avoid eating out unless it is a special occasion with others. Restaurants cook with a large amount of oil and salt. I cannot know exactly what is in the food in a restaurant, so I am eating blindly. I plan my day and take food from home if possible. I travel for work constantly and find a grocery store with prepared salads and a bakery instead of going to a restaurant if at all possible.

I first take out the crackers, chips, and cookies from a client's diet. These are full of empty salt, sugar, and carbohydrates that don't have nutritional value, making you consume them mindlessly. Salt and sugar snacks are addictive snack ingredients. This would be a week-one adjustment. I never make more than one adjustment in someone's diet per week. Notice, I do not discuss calories with the client.

For the second week, I usually don't make actual food changes, letting them adjust, but I make them look at their eating habits. *Are you eating in front of the television or computer? Are you eating in the car?* This is also mindless eating. Eat at a table with other people or just quietly alone. Don't eat while scrolling through your phone. Concentrate on your food.

I point out the carbohydrates in someone's diet. I make the suggestion we only consume the carbohydrates during lunchtime and not dinner time. We need carbohydrates to move our bodies, not to sleep. This small adjustment gets my clients to think about food as fuel for the body. Understand that the carbohydrates that we overlook (such as rice, potatoes, and bread) all add calories we may not need every day. All of these carbohydrates become sugar in your bloodstream and cause ups and downs in energy levels. I see clients from 7:00 a.m. to 7:30 p.m. I need to be at the same energy level throughout the day. I can't have sugar spikes in my bloodstream caused by carbohydrates.

In the third week, my client usually misses their absentminded snacking habit. I ask them to change what they snack on. We add nuts or small fruits, like raspberries, that have that snacking feel and can only be consumed in small quantities. Take the amount of nuts or fruit, put it on a plate so that you can see all of it, then just eat and savor it. Don't do anything else. This is not a time issue. Eating a small snack will take less than three minutes, and you know you have that time. Frozen blueberries and grapes also work well as snacks. Don't snack in front of your work computer.

In the fourth week, I take the carbohydrates completely out of dinner. Carbohydrates break down into sugar readily available to the brain and body for fuel. We are just going to sleep and don't need fuel; we need to rest. I prescribe protein and vegetables for dinner, then ask my clients to consider what they add to those dishes. Good fats, like butter, are great because they satisfy our bodily needs. Sugar in BBQ sauces, prepared oils, and salad dressings add huge amounts of calories. Can they learn to cook without them, using an acid, like vinegar or lemon juice, and spices?

After this simple adjustment, all of my clients lose weight without counting any calories and without completely changing their current habits. Now, I want all of my clients to focus on what drives them to eat. Is it actually hunger? Do they really need to eat breakfast? If they sit at a computer for work, then maybe not. Maybe some coffee and some cantaloupe are good enough in the morning. Or maybe they don't need to eat lunch. Maybe they can eat around 10:00 a.m., then again around 6:00 p.m. Now, in the second month, we figure out what they need mealtime-wise and work on those adjustments.

I would also like to add some simple ideas. I buy most of my vegetables prepared in bags in the fresh produce aisle—bags of broccoli, salad bags, premade salsa (pico de gallo). I buy frozen unbreaded fish packs from the frozen section. This way, I can make my dinners quickly when I get home from work.

Making small adjustments to mindset and food preparation can change the way we eat for the rest of our lives. I don't need to think about calories or what I can or can't eat. I enjoy my food and what it does for my body.

Most clients find after two to three months, the cravings for salty and sugary snacks go away. They can have a small amount now and not want more.

Very important not to beat yourself up when you find yourself eating because you are mentally upset. All of us will binge eat or drink to satisfy some mental issue. Get through it and move on. If it happens often, then the cause of stress needs to be addressed. Even I have eaten a whole box of See's Candy after a bad relationship breakup, though. (Yeah, he wasn't worth it.)

If any one of the first four needs—water, shelter, sleep, or food—gets out of balance, then we can't do the one thing our body needs the most of: exercise.

### EXERCISE

In this book, I have included a few exercises anyone can do at home. I also have videos, live classes you can join, and in-person classes. But I want to start off with some simple concepts about exercise.

Your body was made to move. Watch a three-year-old child. They constantly run around and laugh. Try to keep them still, and they cry or scowl. They laugh because their blood is pumping and it feels good to move. Why do so many people run 5Ks on Thanksgiving? Just stand at the end of a race and watch the smiling faces. They run because the human body loves to move, even if moving is sometimes a struggle. Now exercise doesn't have to be something you hate. Find something you love. And keep trying different sports until you find the body movement you love.

When contemplating what type of exercise to do, the first question I ask a client is, Do you like to exercise alone or with others? If you want to be around others, play golf or tennis, join a running group, or enlist a workout buddy to motivate yourself. Just try things out, and be honest with yourself. I am a loner, so I prefer running alone, but I love the camaraderie of racing. Find your comfort zone. Some people hate competition. l love it. You don't need to compete to play a sport. Find what works for you.

If exercise is not part of your daily routine, don't make it tough. Just exercise for ten minutes a day. Go for a walk, garden, stretch, or do a workout video. Make this a priority for your day, and build it up. The average person needs to exercise for thirty to sixty minutes a day, five days a week, for optimum health. When you meet my clients in the upcoming chapters, you will see how I incorporate exercise into their daily lives. We figure out the types of exercises they enjoy (singular or group) and when it is convenient to exercise. The most important part of exercise is to make it fun, just like you are that three-year-old running around the yard laughing, like you are a child again.

# CHAPTER 8

# LET'S START MOVING!

I have a rule of thumb no matter who the client is; it doesn't matter if it is a teenager running a fast mile on his high school track team or a three-hundred-pound woman trying to lose weight. I don't give a client more than they can do!

My job as a personal trainer is to instruct my clients to move without pain or injury. I need to convince them that exercise will move them to the place they want to be, safely both emotionally and physically.

Everyone needs these things to start their fitness programs:

1. A heart rate monitoring watch. Our heart is a pump, and we need to know how it is working and how to

make it work better. Most people have no idea how their heart works, so this is why I suggest everyone wear a heart rate watch all day, every day, as much as they can. Our hearts don't only work when we are exercising; they work when we sleep, when we argue at work, and every other moment. It is important to know what makes your heart rate spike and what is good for you—and what is not.

2. A great pair of shoes. Sore feet are the worst! If your feet hurt, you won't want to work out. Invest in a good pair of athletic shoes. Go to a running shop that can fit you properly, but don't let them oversell you. Any good running shop should have a treadmill, so they can see how you move. Some can make computer readouts of what your feet look like. It is so worth the money and time to get properly fitted for athletic shoes.

3. Time. One hour a day is four percent of your day. I get lots of calls from prospective clients who want to work out at 7:00 or 8:00 at night, after they finish their twelve-hour workday. Are you kidding me? How effective will your workout be when you are exhausted, hungry, and want to watch TV and go to bed? I stopped taking clients that late in the evening. I also stopped taking clients who want to work out at 6:00 a.m. when they usually don't get up until 7:00 or 8:00 a.m. These clients are sleepy and not engaged. If you can't put in

one hour a day for your health, figure out what times of day work best, or make that commitment, paying me to work out with you is useless.

Same as you did with your sleep survey, figure out what times work out best and dedicate yourself to getting exercise in that time frame as often as you can. Yes, it will take sacrifice, maybe less screen time or less whatever, and life will get in the way, but this is so important; and if your health isn't worth it, then again, the motivation is missing. Find the commitment. I work out with most of my clients two to three times a week and suggest they get a total of five hours of exercise a week. In the beginning, I always suggest two days of working out in a row, then one day rest. This can be modified to fit your schedule, but the body does need rest. I rarely suggest, even for myself, more than four days in a row of exercise. Now an off-day from exercise doesn't mean just eating chocolate and sleeping. An off-day means being active, such as walking or hiking, just not as intensely as your regular workouts.

4. Trust and a positive attitude. Trust that if you put in the time and effort, you will succeed. If you have always hated the idea of exercise, you won't put in the effort, and you will fail. Make yourself try with an open mind. Just try, and I promise you, the results will be amazing.

## A TYPICAL FORTY-FIVE-TO-SIXTY-MINUTE WORKOUT WITH ME IN THE STUDIO

From wheelchair users to fast runners, all my clients work out in this one-hour time frame I recommend, but please adjust this to your needs and availability:

**Five Minutes:** Start with a warm-up.

Move your joints around, slowly in circular motions—hips, ankles, knees, nothing fast and nothing jerky. Arm circles. Just movement. Feel your body: are your ligaments popping, or are your joints making strange, cracking noises? Acknowledge this pain and try to work out of it. Don't move until you're in pain; move to make your current pain diminish and your body loosen.

This is question time for my clients: "How are you feeling? Your knee looks wobbly. Did you sleep well this weekend?" Most people really don't know how their bodies feel and ignore them. I try to get my clients to pay attention to their bodies.

**Five Minutes:** Get the heart moving.

Do medium-pace movements with your arms while moving your legs to get your circulation up and moving through your body. Start to try to listen to your breath. Can you make it rhythmic, and can you feel the difference when your heart is beating fast compared to slowly? Do you know your resting heart rate? What happens to your heart rate when you move? Feel it.

Move your arms up and down over your head while doing a slight jog, small jumping jacks, shallow lunges back and forth and side to side with your arms moving also.

Pay attention to your body. Where is it stiff? Are you getting tired too easily. Do you need to modify this warm-up, as in slow down, to make it more comfortable?

**Thirty Minutes:** On your feet. Weight work and jumping.

**Fifteen Minutes:** Mat work. Flexibility and core work.

**Five Minutes:** Cool down and stretch. We do static stretching at the end.

You should feel tired but energized toward the end of your workout! Drink lots of water and shower. Showering as soon as possible will keep you from getting chilled from the sweat on your skin and prevent bacteria from forming.

On the next few pages, I have given you some common exercises I do with my clients with ideas on how to modify them to fit your abilities. These are just starting points to move your body.

No one starts off doing any exercises perfectly. I don't give exact repetitions or give my clients a number when we start off an exercise. This is because I work off the principle that you do an exercise until you start to get tired or it gets difficult, and you go twenty percent past that level. As an example, if you are doing push-ups and they seem impossible and difficult at eight, then I would have you do two more for a total of ten. This builds muscle and endurance plus the feeling of accomplishment by doing more than you thought you could.

Exercise shouldn't always be hard and should never be painful. Try to make whatever exercise program you do be fun and enjoyable so you will want to continue to do it.

You can find exercise videos on my YouTube Channel[1] and on Recess.tv.[2]

---

1  Vanessa Bogenholm, Fitness 23 Vanessa Bogenholm, YouTube (2020–2021). https://www.youtube.com/channel/UCrsWdWONp7J2EgVQZjtae4g.
2  Vanessa Bogenholm, Vanessa@Fitness23, Recess.tv. (2021). https://recess .tv/@Vanessa_Fitness23.

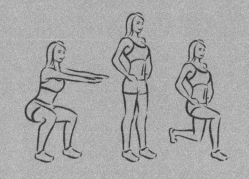

# *EXERCISES*

# *WALKING*

Incorporate walking into your life. Park your car at the end of the parking lot. Take walk breaks while you are working at your desk job.

Walking is a great exercise for everybody to do every day. I even have my overweight clients set aside time to walk for ten minutes every day. Stay erect with your shoulders back, arms flowing freely, landing lightly on your feet.

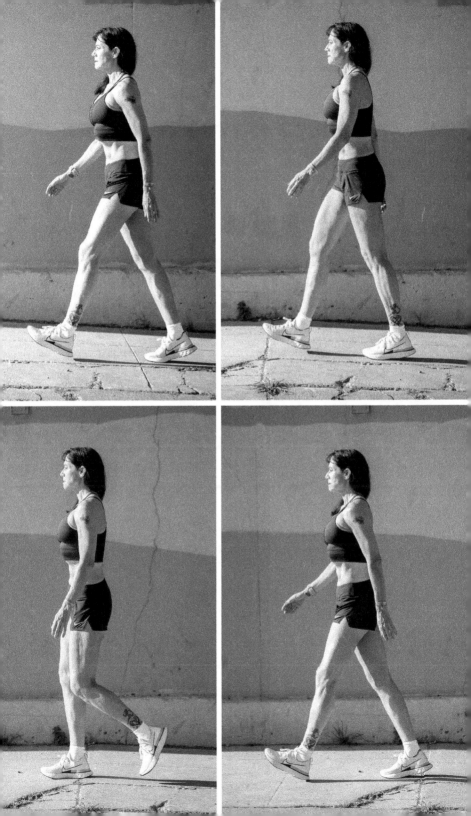

# WEIGHT AND LEG EXTENSIONS

This is a great exercise for working on balance and lengthening and contracting your muscles.

This is a full body workout. Stretch out your arms in one direction with your opposite leg going in the other direction. Bring the arms and leg back to your center core, balancing on your other leg.

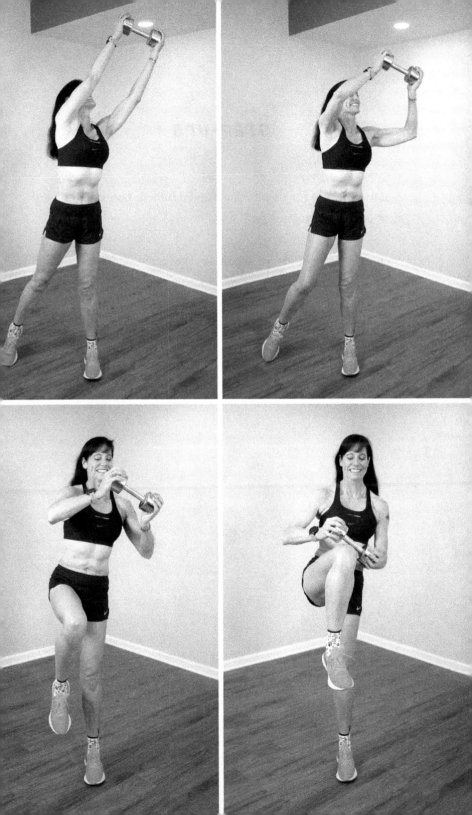

# *STEP-UPS*

A starting point for this exercise could be a step in your house next to a wall for security.

Step-ups can be done anywhere at any height with or without hand weights. Going up on one foot is a great balancing exercise. This exercise is good for your back, core, and legs. It is a great all-over body exercise.

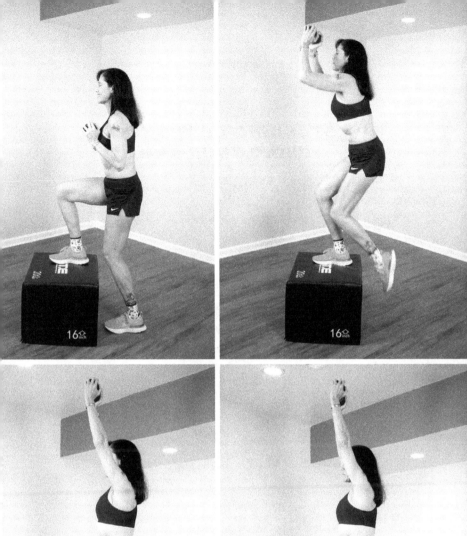

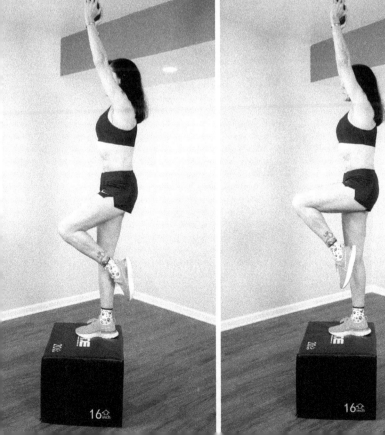

# STANDING UP WITHOUT USING YOUR ARMS

This is a necessary exercise, especially as we age.

Sounds simple, but many people can't do this completely off a chair or bench. Don't lean forwards or sideways. Instead, use mid-thigh to get up. Get as straight as you can at the top to work your back and improve your posture. When you are straight, your ears should be over your ankles.

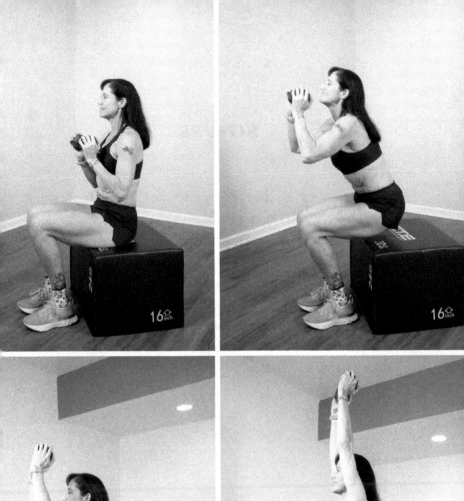

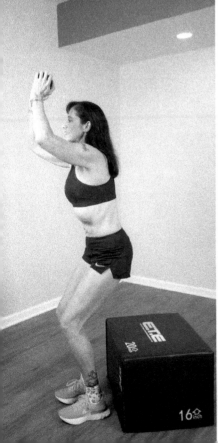

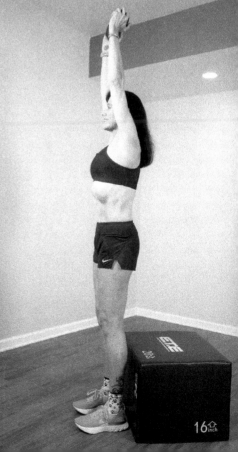

# SIT-UPS

Sit-ups are a great exercise for your core and back. In the beginning, your core won't know how to engage. Your back will strain. As you do more, your stomach muscles will take over.

Definitely one of my favorite exercises. In my studio, most clients do thirty-five sit-ups. It's kind of our tradition. Notice feet are flat on the mat, working your calf at the same time. If getting up from the mat is difficult, put a pillow behind your back or use weights for leverage.

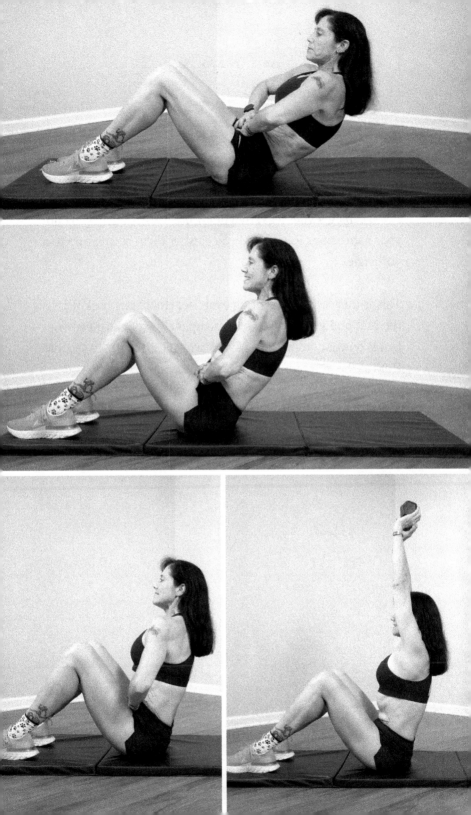

# STRAIGHT LEG RAISE

Tight hamstrings cause back pain by pulling on the lower back. If you can't get your legs straight up, use a wall to help you until your hamstrings loosen and you can get them straight up to a 90° angle.

This is a back and hamstring exercise. Hold your back flat on the mat and get those legs up completely straight. Keep your hands on your stomach to push down your back flat to the mat. Hold at the different levels for thirty seconds.

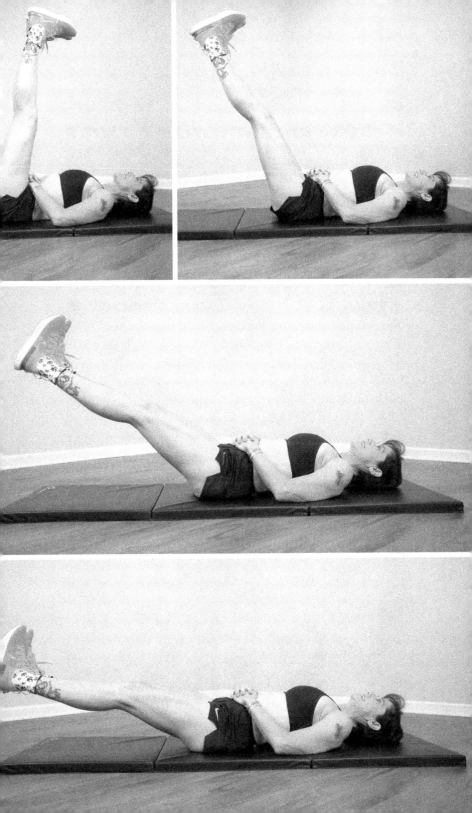

# CORE BALANCE WITH A TWIST

Everyone wants a tight, small waist and a back without pain. This takes work. If this exercise is difficult, do it in stages (one leg up at a time, just five seconds, etc.).

Balance on your butt, using your core to hold your legs and upper body up off the mat. Adding a twist to each side fires up the obliques and raises the difficulty of the exercise.

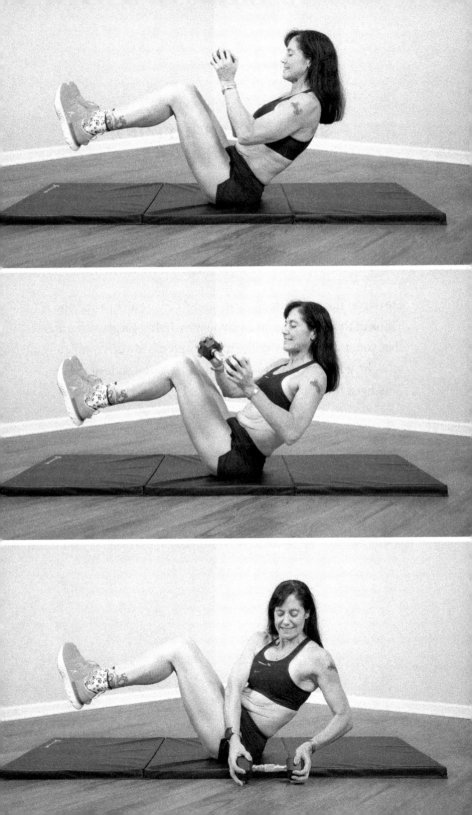

# SIT-UP WITH A TWIST, LEGS STRAIGHT

Lying down and getting back up requires back and core strength when you don't use your arms to push up. This is necessary for getting out of bed without hurting yourself.

Lie flat on the mat with one arm straight in the air at a 90° angle. Think of the arm in the air as if you were holding a glass of water that you don't want to spill. Sit your upper body up completely straight, adding a twist to either the left or right side at the end. This twist fires up your obliques for a tighter twist.

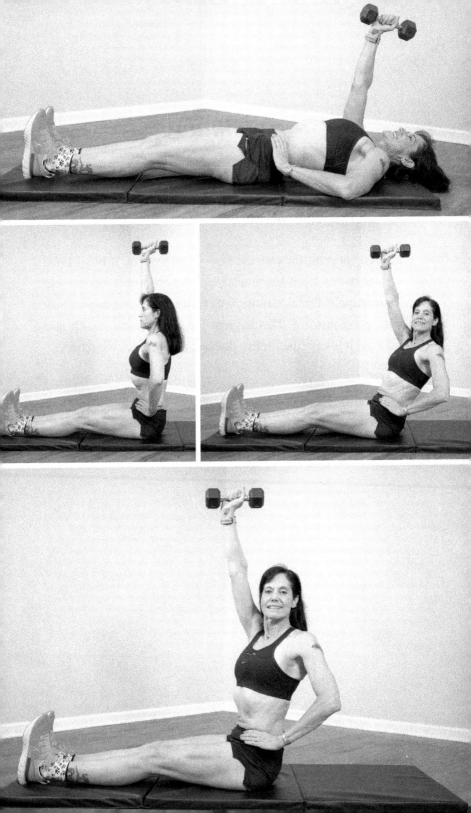

# *RUNNING*

I have been a runner since I was thirteen years old. I still don't know if I get more out of running mentally or physically.

Running is great for your cardiovascular system. It helps build strong bones from the impact on the ground, keeping your joints supple. Practice running as softly as you can on your feet with good posture. This is great for your mental health also because it is very meditative due to the repetitive movement.

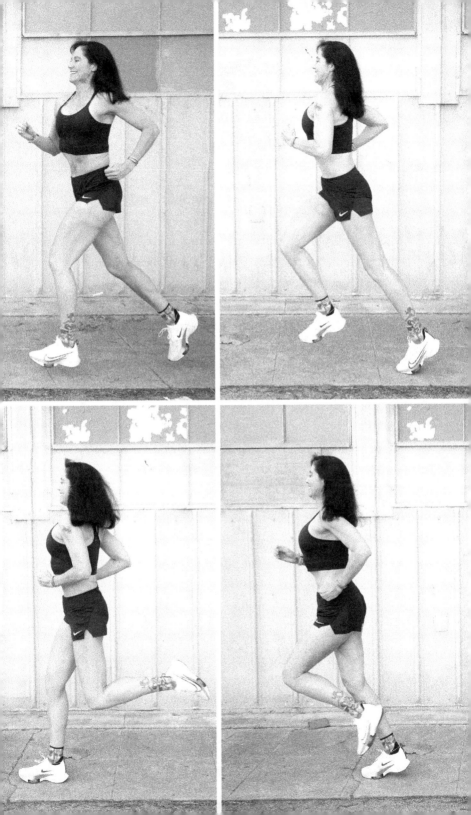

# PUSH-UPS

I use push-ups for everyone of all ages and body types.

Push-ups are a great arm and core workout, improving your overall body strength. If your arms and back are not strong enough, put a pillow under your abdomen so that you are only going down half-way. This will help you keep the correct form with a flat back until you are strong enough to do a full push-up.

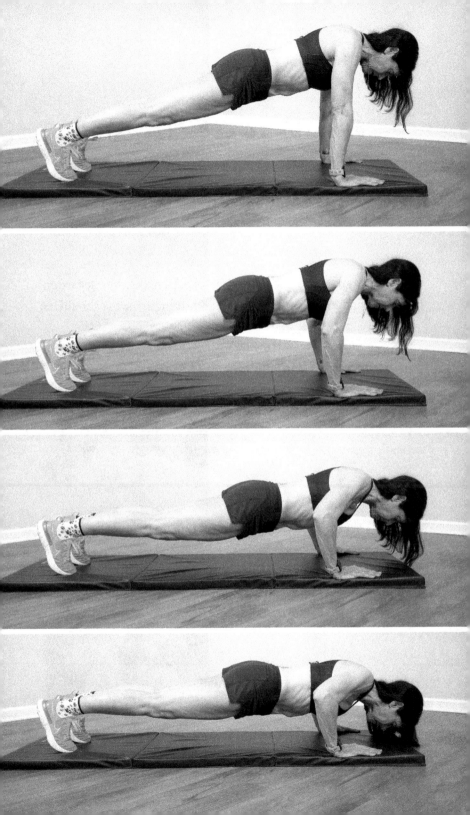

## *PUSH-UP TO LEG EXTENSION*

Being in the up position of a push-up is a great overall exercise for the body. Use a pillow if necessary to start holding up your body.

This is a great exercise to get that long, lean look. The leg extension lengthens the back muscles and strengthens the shoulders.

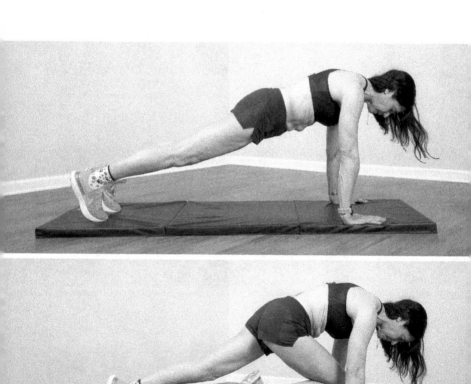

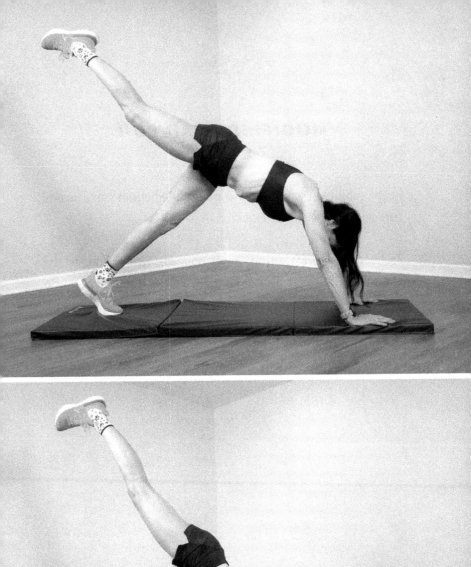
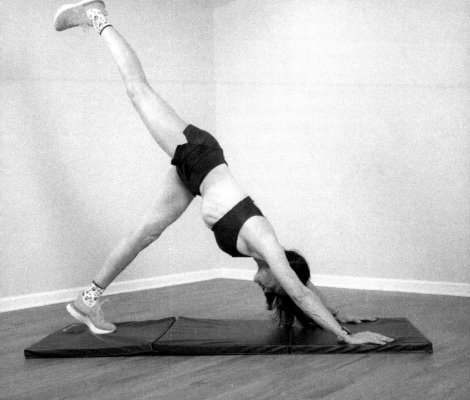

# MODIFIED DEAD BUG

Keep mobility in your legs and arms while building up a strong core and back with this exercise.

From the upright position, lower opposite arm and leg to the mat and raise them back up slowly. This is a great core, arm, and leg exercise.

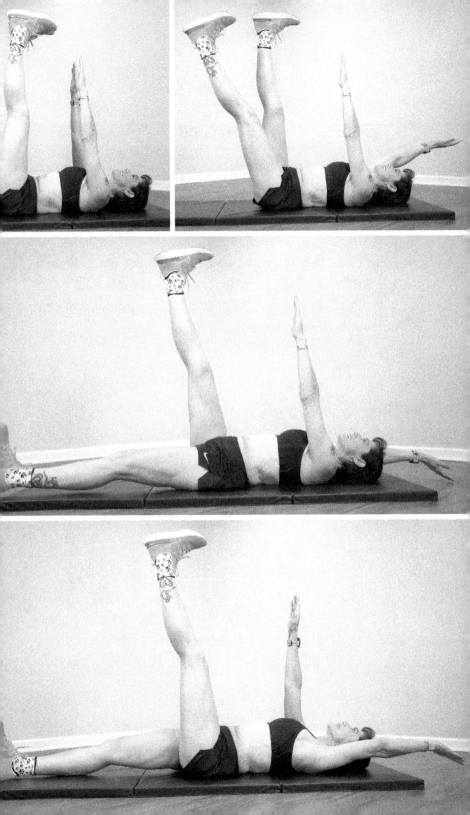

# *LUNGES*

As we age, kneeling down can become more difficult due to lack of use of our legs, from knee injuries, weight issues, etc.

Lunges are always a great exercise for posture, legs, and back strength. Weights can be added for strong shoulders and adds difficulty to the exercise. If this is difficult or painful, don't go down as far or use a step.

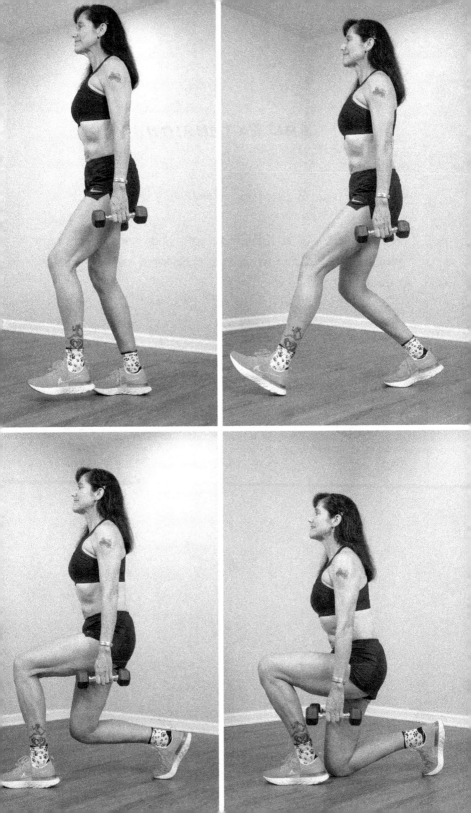

# ARM EXTENSIONS

Strong arms aid in daily living at any age.

Hold an arm out straight from your body with or without weights. This exercise works your back, arms, and rib cage. Be careful not to strain your neck.

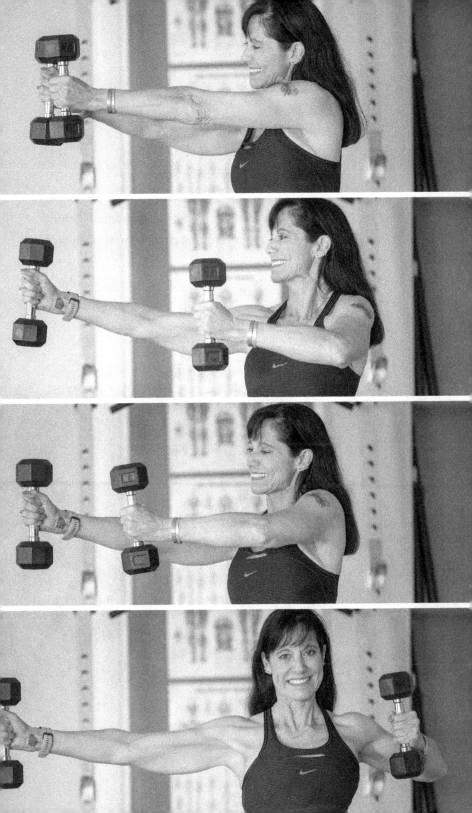

# *BICEP CURL AND SHOULDER PUSH*

Everyone wants and needs strong-looking shoulders. Strong shoulders also help the upper back and neck from being in pain.

Both of these exercises create strong upper arms and shoulders. Keep a straight back during the exercises, engaging your core.

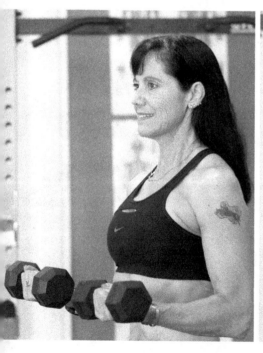
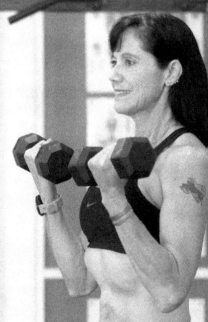

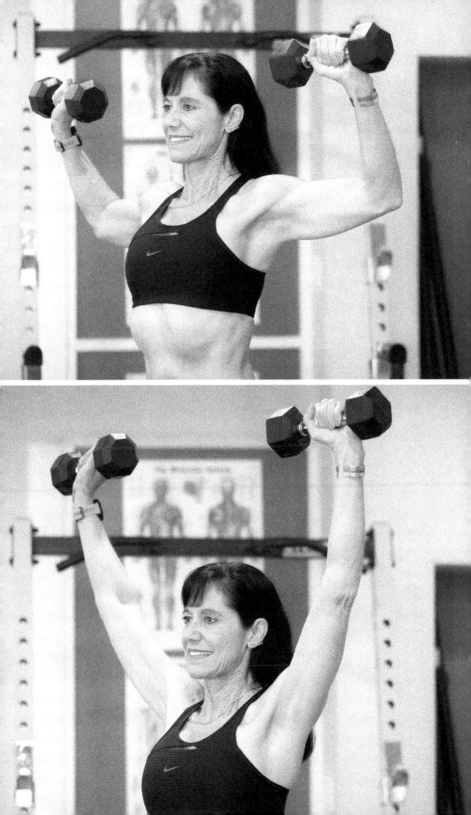

# *JUMPING*

Jump to a level that is comfortable. This could be just two inches. Even small jumps are a big effort and good exercise.

I am such a big believer in jumping. Great overall exercise for legs, body, and strength. Jumping also builds strong bones and strengthens the muscles of the pelvic floor.

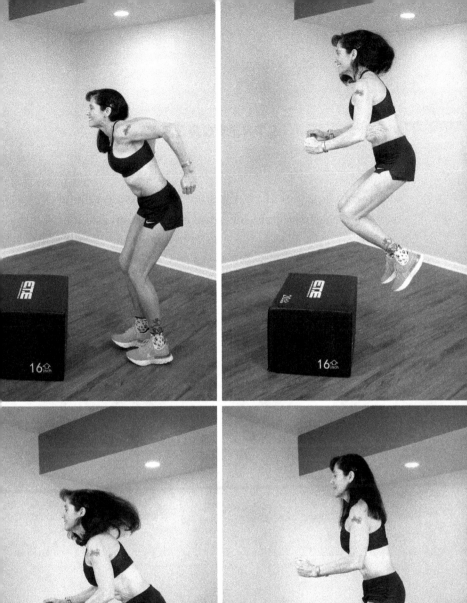

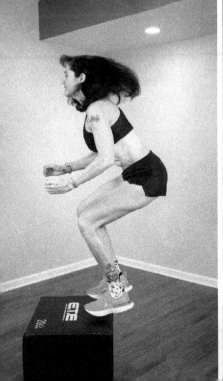

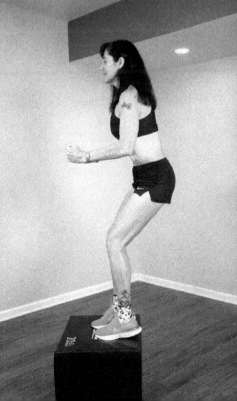

## STRETCHES

Make stretching part of your routine for at least 10 minutes a day. Make sure to stretch your arms, core, back, and shoulders.

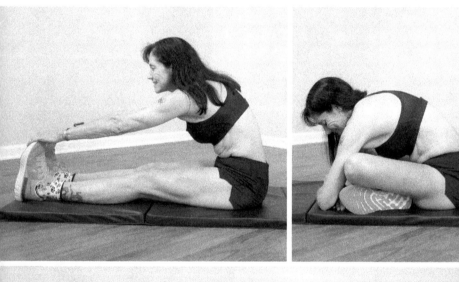

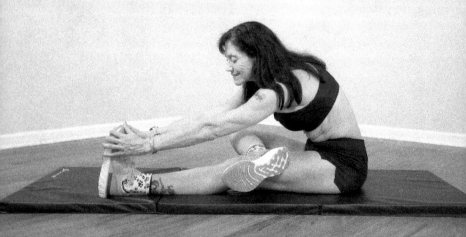

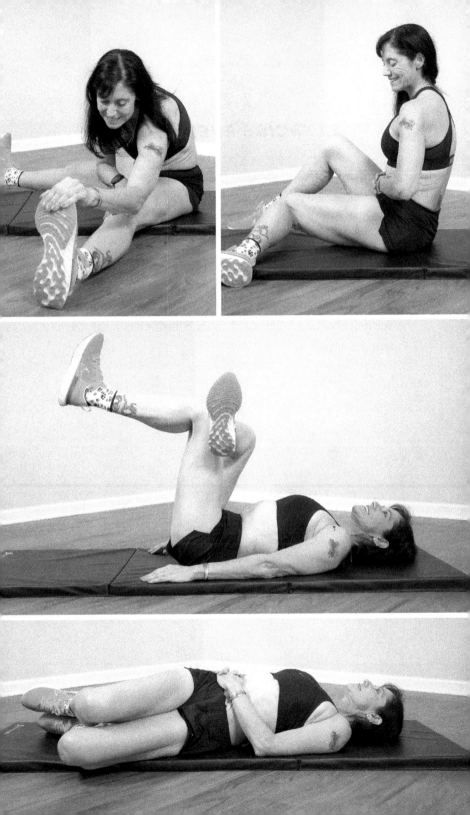

# EXERCISE EVERYWHERE

Our lives are busy. Sometimes just going to a gym or exercise class just isn't possible. And of course, not everyone wants to run for an hour!

Learn to incorporate exercise wherever you are in your daily life. This can be done in between calls in the office or just in your neighborhood. Being out in the sunshine is great for your mental health.

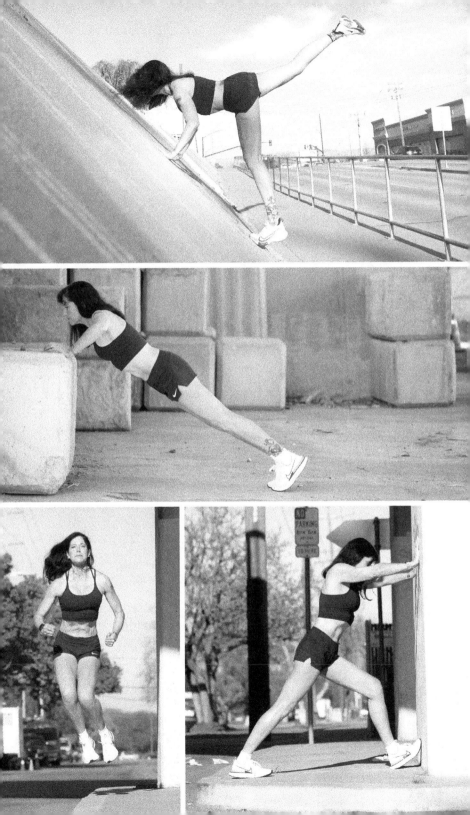

# PART 3

# LET'S MEET SOME REAL PEOPLE

# CHAPTER 9

# PEOPLE ARE DIFFERENT. MY APPROACHES ARE DIFFERENT TOO.

E nough about me! Let's meet some real clients and follow them on their fitness journeys to enjoying their bodies. In the following chapters, I will discuss real people, and I hope you find inspiration in their stories.

Please note all stories of individuals have their first names changed to protect their privacy. The only real first name I use is a man named Jack who has since passed away. This book is dedicated to him. Without him, my personal training career would not have been possible.

I always laugh at books, articles, and videos showing a one-size-fits-all approach to getting healthy and feeling good about your body. I have never seen two people that act alike, look alike or feel alike, so why would my approach to my 10:00 a.m. twenty-two-year-old female client look similar to my 5:00 p.m. seventy-five-year-old male client?

Everyone comes to me with different problems, wishes, physical, and mental abilities. In the next few chapters, I hope the people I have worked with inspire you. These clients worked hard to improve their bodies, achieve realistic and long-lasting success, be pain-free, and feel better physically (which translates to less mental stress).

I have grouped people by the reasons they sought me out as a personal trainer by giving examples of types of people. My clients will recognize themselves as they walked in the door and first started with me. They will remember the hard work they put in through the years, the ups and downs, and the continuing work they continue to do in their lives, both in and out of the gym, to achieve long-term success mentally and physically.

Many of these stories will be raw and painful. I haven't always succeeded in helping people. In fact, you are going to read about suicide, death, and hospitalizations in these chapters. You will feel the pain and the tears and the frustrations people have with their bodies.

But you will also hear about overwhelming success against all odds. I hope to express the joy of a man losing one hundred twenty-eight pounds and going on his first date in twenty years (She asked him out!); the amazement when Jack (the only real name I use in this book) got out of his wheelchair and walked down the hall with his walker for the first time; and the tears of a boy who had never been athletic, breaking five minutes per mile for the first time at a track meet, becoming the star on his high school team, and getting a full ride running scholarship to college.

Every day, I see seven to twelve people who just want to feel better, and I feel blessed that they have asked me for help. I will try to do their stories justice.

*CHAPTER 10*

# HOW I APPROACH WORKING WITH A NEW CLIENT

C lients come to me through a referral from another client or by finding me on an internet search, seeing me at a running race, or driving by and seeing my studio in San Jose, CA.

All of my clients are suspicious of me in the beginning. They come in slightly scared, embarrassed, and either don't want to commit or are overzealous with starting an exercise program. I always say when someone first starts their personal training journey with me, "We are going to spend lots of time together, two to three hours a week, so if you don't like me or I don't like you for any reason, this isn't going to work—and no hard feelings. I just want what is best for you." And this is the truth. I see the pain in everyone, and I want that pain alleviated, whether I can help the person or not.

Most of the clients want to know what we are going to do exercise-wise and what kind of diet are they going on. Honestly, I don't really know when I first meet a client. I want to get quiet with them, listen to how they view themselves and their bodies, see what kind of family and work life they have, help them map their goals, and gauge how hard they can physically and mentally work. The best and most often asked question by new clients is, "How long is this going to take, three months, a year, what do you think? When will I look and feel better?"

None of my clients want to hear the honest answer to this question. Everyone is looking for an easy quick fix to life. The true answer is, "This process will take the rest of your life." But most clients aren't ready and don't want to hear that in the first week with me, so I refrain from saying it. Usually, I just smile and let it go. I tell them the truth. If they try, they will see positive changes in three weeks which will build with time to where they want to be with their bodies.

I don't give any free workout sessions. I let a client meet me, talk to me for about twenty minutes in person or on the phone and see the facility for a few minutes so they understand the general process, but that is it. The client has to book and pay for at least one session. I have found this "buy-in" makes them show up and seriously consider this life change. At the end of that first session, I ask if they would like to continue, and we talk finances and time constraints. We can do one hour a week or two or three hours per week, depending on their time and financial abilities. I give the same effort for every client whether they do one or three hours per week.

When someone walks in the door, I immediately begin to analyze their posture and pain levels. I ask them about body injuries (past and current), current medications, (even over the counter), and sleep patterns. I ask questions about their lives, families, and work while instructing them through simple warm-up exercises, so they are distracted. This technique allows the client to relax while I contemplate their physical abilities and mental state. I pay attention to their heart rate and breathing. Shoulder, knee, back, and hip issues are common with everyone, and the first thing I always do is try to straighten their posture and have them realize how crooked their body is and feel it, feel their bodies. Feel the difference from their left and right sides as they move. I want the client to determine their balance, strength or weakness, which side of their body feels better than the other—to feel all of it, not just see it in a mirror. I have a large mirror in the studio but refrain from using it. I find that most people, especially those experiencing pain or discontentment, don't know how to feel their bodies. Many clients have chosen to ignore their bodies as much as possible.

I will try to be gentle here, and please don't see this as judgmental. Almost ninety percent of my clients lied to me during our first five to ten personal training hours spent together. They don't mean to lie. I think it is human nature, or a human coping mechanism, to lie to ourselves and others to make ourselves feel better.

Most clients will lie about their weight, workout patterns, medications, and pain levels. The scale for weight and body fat is in the bathroom, completely private, and doesn't record anything. I encourage clients to use it weekly, but they don't have to tell me what it says. I will ask them, in passing, but never want to see the proof for the first few months. I never confront someone on a lie. I used to lie to myself often when I was younger because I was so unhappy. I just hope a client's lies will dissipate as they become more comfortable with me.

When I am working with clients on significant weight loss, their weight will fluctuate. I ask long-term clients to get on the scale, so I can keep track and move them forward accordingly. Sometimes they look at the scale, and sometimes they don't, but I need to keep them moving forward, so I record their weight.

Does the client understand their body rhythm? Most just look at me and shrug when I ask this question. Everyone has a timetable and a time of day that works better for them to exercise and sleep, but very few people pay attention to this rhythm or body clock. I am an early morning runner. 4:30 a.m. is kind of my wheelhouse. Ask me to run at 5:00 p.m., and I would rather have a vodka tonic and a nap hanging out with my dogs. We all have work, families, school, etc. I also have a full work schedule, but if you are a morning person trying to make yourself work out at night because of your work schedule or a timeslot I have open, that is a recipe for failure. Understanding your body clock allows you to set yourself up to succeed with your body goals.

No major changes should happen in the first few workouts, and the client should never hurt. You might be sore after a workout, but there should never be sharp long-lasting pain. Soreness is worse two days after a workout, so I get the client ready to experience that delayed soreness. We try to build flexibility, strength, cardio, good posture, and balance into all workouts whether the client is eighty-six years old and just trying to stay mobile, one hundred pounds overweight, or training for sports.

No major dietary changes to start. I structure dietary changes to fit the client's needs. I want them to understand food as a tool that enables them to do what they want to do for their own happiness. The client has to learn to feel their bodies and the consequences food choices have on their preferred activities (even if the activity is just going to sleep, as it too is affected by our food choices).

The only dietary change I add for everyone immediately is: drink water every day. Plain water. Thirty to forty ounces in the morning, thirty to forty ounces again around 3:00 p.m. Chug it down! This easy daily addition controls common dehydration. Most clients are open to this for the first three days, then it becomes work to drink this much water. Clients have a difficult time sticking to the water regime even if it makes them feel better. It usually takes over two months for this amount of water to become a habit for the client to do without resistance.

Many clients tell me they hate water and don't want to drink water at all. They want to drink alcohol, coffee, tea, or soft drinks instead and think it should do the same thing for their bodies. This becomes a difficult situation for me. Caffeine, alcohol, and diet drinks all cause dehydration. These drinks can also hurt your kidneys and liver. I try to be patient, but when a client won't even drink water, they won't stick to any diet or exercise program I suggest. Change is difficult for most people. I have many clients that have had headaches, skin conditions, kidney stones, and gastrointestinal problems their entire lives from the lack of drinking water. The client knows they have these problems caused by their lack of a good diet and not drinking water and still won't change. Energy drinks are becoming more common than ever, especially with people under the age of thirty. This dependence on caffeine and sugar is difficult to break and needs to be addressed immediately. I try to get all of my clients off these energy drinks immediately.

I need to digress here and tell a story about the extreme drinking of sodas. I was at a wine festival on a blind date that wasn't going well (most of my dates don't go well, but that is for another book). A couple in their mid-sixties, well dressed and dignified looking, stopped me and asked if they could speak to me. I said "of course" with a smile. They had heard of me from a friend, thought of calling me on the phone but chickened out. They recognized me from my pictures on my website. They looked at each other uneasily as they spoke. The mother took the lead to tell me what she needed to say. Their daughter was a shut-in house bound thirty-year-old. She was college educated at an Ivy League school and, by her parents' guess, at least one hundred pounds overweight. Could I help their daughter? My date was aghast at what these people were telling me, a total stranger, about their daughter in public.

"What kind of personal trainer are you?" he asked right in front of the girl's parents.

I told my date to leave immediately, so I could talk to the parents privately. The mother was blaming herself for Marybeth's obesity and life status and started crying. The father wouldn't even look at me. He kept looking at the crowd walking by as if he was no longer listening to the conversation between me and his wife. I felt their pain as if it was my own. I know the pain of obesity too well. I agreed to come to their home and meet Marybeth the following evening.

Marybeth, who was close to three hundred and fifty pounds, tried to be shocking to me: rude, demanding, mean. She drank eight cans of ginger ale a day. She refused to budge on this sugar consumption. I suggested she only drink four ginger ales a day, watering down the cans with water. I tried. I didn't push and moved on to other discussions. In this first meeting, her mother fussed over her daughter, embarrassed at their home life. The father stayed slightly out of vision in the kitchen. I could hear him walking around. I asked the mother to leave the room so I could work out her daughter. I got Marybeth off of the couch and moving. She laughed at my stand-up comedy routine. Within thirty minutes of her mom leaving the room, she admitted to me why this overweight locked-in situation had happened. Her first love in college had dumped her seven years earlier and she just started eating and didn't stop. Marybeth got comfort in food, mental and physical comfort. She didn't want to get better physically. She liked eating. Marybeth admitted she liked having her parents take care of her and hiding from the world by never leaving the house. Her life revolving around online writing and talking to strangers in chatrooms is the life story she shared with me.

My take on her was that she was brilliant. You could just tell the way she spoke. Marybeth had an Ivy League education, wealthy parents, and a full life ahead of her. She was very angry. I agreed to work with her three times a week. She smiled when I was leaving that first day. I felt good too. I thought I had broken through a little and could definitely help her. But I turned around before I left and pushed a little. "How about you water down those ginger ales with a *fourth* of water, just a couple of them?"

"Vanessa, I think I can do that," she replied, pretending as if she was making a huge sacrifice. We both laughed at her drama. We had established a good connection.

I worked with her for a little over a month. The first couple of weeks we were always in the living room of her parents' home, and I would have to ask the mother to leave us alone and not watch us exercising. We worked out late in the evenings because Marybeth didn't even wake up and get out of bed until noon. Because it was dark outside and no one could see her, I convinced her to go out on the back patio. Then I convinced her to walk with me outside. At a month in, she could now walk around the block with me, and I heard her laugh many times, and it was delightful. Marybeth lost twenty pounds in that first month, sweating and cursing and laughing.

Her brother came home for a family visit. Her mother canceled the weekend appointment since her son was home and the family was spending time together.

Marybeth had a violent mental breakdown with her brother over family money that weekend. The police came and arrested her. To avoid serious jail time, Marybeth was committed to a mental hospital. I never saw her again. Her father cried when he came to my studio to hand me a check and say thank you. "My daughter laughed more with you than we had heard for years...I hope you will work with her again when she gets out." It has been three years since I saw her. Marybeth is still in a mental facility.

Let's get back to hydration and me working with a new client. It is easy to fall out of habits, even if they are good habits. I will still need to remind my clients occasionally of the necessity to stay hydrated for years.

My goals with a new client are rarely what they tell me are their goals in these first sessions. I usually notice long-time imbalances and structural problems. I point these out to the client, so they can begin to understand their bodies. My goal is to get them moving, feeling better and happy at the end of every session. Everyone should feel better after a workout session. Stronger, more flexible, and mentally happier.

I never give timetable goals. Clients are always looking for how long I think something, like getting a shoulder to work again, lose twenty pounds, etc. will take. I have no idea. Humans aren't machines. Patience must happen, and acceptance of the work needing to take place plus sacrifices to make the body they want and deserve.

Heart rate is so important. Most people don't have a clue what their hearts are doing in their bodies. I always suggest a heart rate monitoring watch. I am a runner and prefer Garmin watches, but Apple watches or any other brand will work. A good watch costs about one hundred and twenty-five dollars, so all of my clients (and most other people) can reasonably afford them.

When clients first get heart rate monitoring watches, they are obsessed with the data. They keep looking at the watch, and I have to tell them to focus on the exercise and try to feel their body and effort. I try to keep the use of this heart rate data simple. The slower your heart beats, the easier your heart is working, so the easier the exercise. The stronger your body, heart and respiration, which have to work together, and the less stress you are putting on your body and mind, the better you feel when you push yourself physically. As long as the client doesn't have any serious medical issues, we shoot for a resting heart rate between fifty-five to seventy beats per minute. When we stand up, our hearts immediately go up fifteen to twenty beats per minute to get our bodies ready to move. Nice easy jogging or fast walking should be one hundred ten to one hundred forty beats per minute (but can fluctuate somewhat based on different factors). This makes running enjoyable. We do faster workouts and run faster in short bursts to build up heart strength. One of the most fascinating things clients learn about their hearts is the stress that mental pain puts on their bodies.

"Oh my god, Vanessa! I was arguing with a guy at work—okay, I was really screaming at him—and my watch started buzzing!" I had told the client to set his watch at a one hundred forty beats per minute alarm for his running. He was new to running, and I didn't want his heart rate to go over one hundred forty for a few weeks. He found out the mental stress of work hurt his heart too because when he was angry, his heart went up over one hundred fifty beats per minute. I just smiled as he told me this. Oh, yeah, he quit that job once he realized the stress was literally killing him.

The last part of starting with a new client is slowing them down mentally and physically. Learning that slow repetition for exercising—be it weights, balance, or endurance like running or bike riding—is the key to almost any goals you want to achieve with your body and mind. I lower the weights, the speed, and the concern. We work toward long-term goals, with short-term monitoring.

As my clients leave these first few workouts with me, they are almost always out the door when they ask, "Oh, so now what do I eat?"

My response: "What does your body tell you it needs after a workout?" Most of them say nothing really, but I loved it when a woman said to me, "You know, Vanessa, yesterday I was craving an orange."

"So, your body was telling you it wanted Vitamin C. Did you eat an orange?" I asked.

"No, I ate a sandwich, it was lunchtime," she responded. "Why did I do that and not listen to what my body was asking for?" I loved this. Here was a client beginning to listen to her body at the age of sixty-eight.

Habits and not paying attention to what our body is asking for, plus the ease of obtaining certain foods, are why we eat what we do and don't consume what our body craves. "Next time eat the orange," I told her smiling.

We need to recognize our habits and move them in directions to make us feel better and get us ready to move our bodies to be the machines we desire to live our best lives.

# CHAPTER 11

# OBESITY

## *WHAT IT REALLY IS AND HOW MUCH IT AFFECTS A PERSON'S LIFE*

Just walk into your local Walmart, Home Depot, Target, or any other large department store and look at the size of the average American. We can argue about why people are obese, but I don't want to go there, yet. I want to address what obesity is and why clients come in to see me and get some help with their obesity problem and how I approach working with an obese client. Obesity, by definition, is a medical condition in which excess body fat has accumulated to the extent that it may hinder your health. It is defined by body mass index (BMI). You can find a free body mass index calculator online. I use the CDC BMI Calculator.

Basically, if your BMI is between twenty-five and twenty-nine, you are overweight, gender notwithstanding. If your BMI is thirty to forty, you are clinically obese, and if your BMI is over forty, you are considered severely obese.

All of the following facts and measurements come directly off of the Centers for Disease Control and Prevention website.

Forty-two-point-four percent of Americans were obese in 2017–2018 according to the Centers for Disease Control and Prevention. According to the World Health Organization, worldwide obesity has tripled since 1975.

From 1999–2000 through 2017–2018, the prevalence of obesity increased from 30.5 percent to 42.4 percent, and the prevalence of severe obesity increased from 4.7 percent to 9.2 percent in the United States.

Obesity-related conditions include heart disease, stroke, type 2 diabetes, and certain types of cancer. These conditions are some of the leading causes of preventable, premature death. Obese people die earlier than people of normal weight. It's just a medical fact. (As I am finishing this book, we are ten months into the Covid pandemic. We know that obese people are dying of this virus more often than people of a regular bodyweight because of the preexisting conditions caused by obesity.)

The estimated annual medical cost of obesity in the United States was $147 billion in 2008; the medical costs for obese people were

$1,429 higher than those of normal weight. Type 2 diabetes is considered the number-one reason for the higher medical bills, with hip, knee, and back issues close behind. Our bodies weren't designed to carry forty, sixty, or even one hundred extra pounds.

Wow, that was very clinical of me. Now let's talk reality.

We have become a very sedentary society. We sit for work. We sit and watch our computers and televisions. We watch sports on TV instead of running around and catching or kicking balls. Most cities aren't made for walking, especially in the United States. Our daily step count is low. Other people do our physical labor. We don't clean our own houses, do our own yard work, work on or wash our own cars. Some people don't even walk their own dogs.

Food is cheap. I didn't say good nutritious food was cheap. You can go into your grocery store and buy fifty tortillas for three dollars. A single cheeseburger at McDonald's is $1.19. A bag of Lay's BBQ chips is $2.50. All of these options are fast, cheap and convenient, offering little to no nutritional value to your body. Consuming these items leaves your body craving even more food to get the nutrients it needs to function properly. This consumption of low-nutrient foods contributes to binge eating. I mean how often have you heard of someone binge eating squash and spinach?

Time is in short supply in many homes with both parents working outside the home, so cooking is difficult. Cooking takes time, and few households cook three full meals a day. Produce goes bad in the refrigerator in a few days if not used, so why buy it if it is too difficult to prepare and no one eats the produce? Drive-through food and delivery are so easy—*let's just get a pizza.* A pizza is fat and carbohydrates and again lacks the nutrients your body craves, so again we overeat trying to satisfy our bodily needs.

We are lonely, bored, etc. so we eat. Eating gives us something to do with our hands and mouths.

Food is used for almost every celebration all around the world and brings us national identity. Birthday cake, Fourth of July BBQ, Sunday night family dinner, Easter ham, Thanksgiving turkey and stuffing, the wedding reception dinner. In Italy, we must eat pasta, perogies in Poland. *Let's celebrate and get some ice cream! Here I bought you some chocolates as a gift.*

We are consuming more alcohol than ever as a society. The average alcoholic drink has one hundred and fifty calories. If you have two drinks a day, that is fourteen drinks a week, and at 3,000-3,500 calories per pound, one pound of fat can come just from alcohol consumption per week. A margarita has about two hundred and fifty calories.

Meat consumption is over two hundred pounds per person in the United States per year. In the 1970s, Americans started choosing beef over chicken to save money, which created many new dietary issues. Beef has three amino acids only found in beef and necessary for humans. Chicken is just protein and does not contain these amino acids, and the poultry associations have spent decades telling consumers it was the healthier option. Chicken is also usually battered and fried adding more empty calories. Restaurants add bacon to nearly everything now, including salads. Bacon contains over fifty percent fat; you can see it on each strip.

Ugh, I feel ready to throw up. Enough. You get the picture. We as Americans are making poor food choices, which mentally and physically lead to obesity.

Everyone has a different breaking point when they realize their weight and obesity are out of control. For some, it is breaking furniture by sitting on it or leaning on it. Especially if this furniture breaks in front of others. For some obese people, being called fat by strangers is a catalyst. For some, it is a health scare like a heart attack. Everyone thinks it is no big deal to carry an extra twenty pounds which then turns into forty pounds then one hundred pounds then—*wow what happened, how did I get this fat?*

Many times, obesity is a family issue. The whole family eats unhealthy food in large amounts and doesn't move. Everyone in the house is obese, and no one in the house tries to break the cycle.

Some sought help from me. Let's meet them.

# CHAPTER 12

# MEET SOME OF MY (FORMERLY) OBESE CLIENTS

*(Fair Warning: Some Are Dead)*

This woman was the second obese client I worked with as a personal trainer. Fair warning: this is a sad story. (Remember, I changed all their names to protect their privacy.)

Alice called me and said she was severely obese and didn't leave her house often. Alice was living in a small cottage behind her parent's home. She asked very politely if I could come to her house to work out with her. I agreed. Alice had received my name from a doctor who did gastric bypass surgery. I had met this doctor at a tennis match, and he told me he could get me some work as I was just starting my personal training business. The doctor wanted her to lose sixty pounds before he performed the weight loss surgery, gastric bypass. Alice was hoping to get the weight loss surgery within the next six months. She was very excited to get the surgery done and move forward with her life. She sounded very upbeat and positive on the phone. I was excited to get her as a client. I loved our energy together on the phone call.

Her parents were extremely wealthy. The house was an estate with a beautiful gate and security system and a cobbled stone driveway going through lush gardens. Her father, an extremely thin man in his seventies, waved me through the gate and pointed out a backhouse for me to drive up to and park. He never spoke to me at any time when I worked with his daughter.

My client was sitting on the couch in her house. Alice was so large she took up most of the couch but still smiled as she pushed herself off the couch in a rolling heaving motion. My guess was she was close to four hundred pounds. Alice was very smiley with a great attitude. She seemed very positive and wanted so much to move forward on this weight loss journey. We did a few exercises. I liked her and agreed to see her four times a week. Alice had a beautiful home with a pool, a private three-hole golf course, beautiful landscaping, and the whole estate was very private. We played basketball, jogged, played soccer, lifted some weights, generally had good productive workout sessions. Alice stayed positive and motivated through-out most of her workout sessions. She was only forty years old, and her joints weren't excessively damaged yet, so she could still move around well even with the extra weight.

The second week I got her on the scale, and she was three hun-dred seventy pounds. Alice didn't look at the scale. She said she didn't want to know how much she really weighed. She just wanted me to report to the doctor when she had lost enough weight for the surgery. We continued working out four days a week. Alice worked very hard, sweating and huffing and puffing and laughing. It took two weeks, but we cleaned out the junk food in her home and bought healthier food. Before that, she ordered all her food through delivery. She did not go shopping in public herself.

When we first met, she couldn't walk for two minutes without sitting down to breathe heavily and rest. Within a month, Alice could walk to the front gate and back in ten minutes. She began walking her dog, a gorgeous Great Dane, every day for at least thirty minutes within two months of us beginning to work out. I was very proud of her hard work.

At the end of the second month, I made her look at the scale. She was down forty-seven pounds. Alice had to keep pulling up her shorts when she worked out; they were now too big. Oh, and she would laugh. Laugh at her attempts at basketball, laugh at her current life, laugh at the prospect of living a full life. She told me of her past and her future. I took her to a local park, the first public place she could be seen by others in over five years, and she walked/jogged with me for thirty minutes.

We were four months into working out together and in a good rhythm. She was now seventy-two pounds down and looked like a different person. I reported her weight loss to the surgeon. I also told him how hard she was working. The doctor was thrilled for her and that I had done so much to help her. I felt good too.

Change came.

I drove to her house one morning, and Alice just looked at me differently. I could feel the change coming, and I knew what she would say before she said it. Alice had decided to quit. All the working out was too much for her, she said. She found an online coach she would work with now. She was dismissing me. I didn't argue; in fact, I didn't say a word. I just got in my car to drive out. She asked for a refund for my services for the week. Alice wanted to use the money for the online service she was now going to use. I told her that since her mother paid me, I would refund her mother. She wanted the money directly, insisting. I refused.

Her mother chased me down the driveway and begged me not to give up on her daughter. I was done too, honestly. I couldn't imagine how someone could work so hard, lose over seventy pounds, and quit on me. This was early in my personal training career. I lacked tolerance and compassion. I was pissed. It was about me, though, not her.

Two months later her mother called me. Alice was in the hospital after having a massive heart attack and was now having quadruple bypass surgery. She had gained sixty pounds back since I had seen her and was again no longer leaving her small house or the property. Would I consider working with her daughter again, Alice's mother asked. I told her to call me when Alice was home from the hospital.

Alice didn't make it home. She died of cardiac arrest at the age of forty-one in the hospital. At the time of her death, she was over three hundred fifty pounds.

Alice was a beautiful, educated woman who ate herself to death. She was the first person I saw die from obesity. I think of her every day. In fact, I think of Alice every time I see an obese woman anywhere. No one should die from eating themselves to death.

A gentleman called me, the phone said it was from a real estate finance company. Earl had lost forty pounds on his own, but seemed to be stuck, unable to lose any more weight. Could I help him? Earl had never really exercised in his life and was now in his mid-fifties. He was very scared of getting hurt doing exercise. He was 5 6 and needed to lose another eighty pounds by his estimation and had scheduled weight loss surgery in three months. He figured it was a good time to start an exercise program, realizing he would need one after the weight loss surgery. He had scheduled the surgery with the same doctor who had referred Alice to me.

In two months of working out with me, Earl had taken off twenty pounds easily. He was exercising with me three times a week and now was bicycling to work every day. We had incorporated exercise into his daily routine and comfortably adjusted his eating habits. He was consuming one thousand one hundred calories a day and realized this was the way he would have to live the rest of his life. He started to smile. When I first met him, he seemed so sad and resigned to live a lonely life.

We had a serious discussion at about three months in. Did I think I could help him get the rest of the weight off without surgery? I did. Earl trusted me and didn't have the weight loss surgery. He lost one hundred twenty-eight pounds in three years and had skin reduction surgery around his waist.

The skin reduction surgery was rough. Surgeons cut off the eight-inch flap of skin Earl used to tuck into his pants, leaving a nine-inch scar across his abdomen. It took over two months to partially close the incision and six months to heal so he could work out fully again. It looked like a Cesarean scar, and we made many jokes about him losing his "baby."

Earl looked amazing. He was a very fit almost sixty-year-old man, happy, and his real estate company was thriving. I met his two adult daughters. They were very encouraging and proud of their father and his weight loss. The love his daughters had for him was beautiful. His daughters had always loved and supported their father. He was the one who cut them out of his life and became distant after his divorce. Earl just thought they would prefer to be around their mother. He had become ashamed of his body and thought his girls didn't love him because he was fat. He was very wrong.

A family wedding was coming up in another state. Earl bought an expensive custom suit because this was the first time he was going to see his ex-wife, who had left him for another man. He hadn't seen her or that side of the family for five years. He was happy and excited to attend this family event and see everyone again.

The ex-wife and everyone else were in shock when they saw Earl at the wedding. When the ex-wife asked him how he lost all the weight, he told her, "Vanessa encouraged me, believed in me, and helped me get healthy." He and his daughters let the ex-wife and everyone at the wedding believe "Vanessa" was a new girlfriend. They loved telling me this story the week after the wedding. It brought them all such joy and was like this little secret with his daughters who loved him so much. We all laughed at this story, but then I told him dating would be good for him. We all deserve a partner. His daughters left, and Earl and I began his workout.

Earl was very quiet after his daughters left. Then he dropped the bomb. "Vanessa, I can't date, my penis doesn't work," he said very matter-of-factly and not the least bit embarrassed.

When you work with clients for two to three hours a week for years, you learn everything about them. He hadn't talked to his doctor about this, but he was willing to tell me. And here is the weirdness of my renaissance life and how a few different careers helped my client. I wrote a fiction book seven years ago. *The Moral Line* is a story of a high-end older escort who falls in love with all of her clients a little and is tackling her own loneliness. During the writing and research of the book, I met many escorts, male and female. I also met a doctor that treated these escorts with respect and kept them healthy.

I told my client, "I got a guy, a doctor, who can help you." Earl made the appointment with the doctor and got the help he needed.

He went on his first date with a woman who asked him out at work. By being asked out, Earl found out he was liked by and attractive to women again. One woman he dated ran away when she found out he had lost over one hundred pounds. One woman kept feeding him, and he gained weight, so that relationship ended too. And yes, he has had sex as a smaller man and said it was "so much more fun to be able to move around!" I told him that was way too much information for this personal trainer. We laughed.

I still hope he will find love, and I see him once a week for his workouts. He is a beautiful soul, and I cry a little every time he walks through the door. Hard work, a little belief, and lots of laughs got him to a better place physically and mentally.

A woman called and asked if I could work with her mother-in-law, who was a "mess and home bound" in a wheelchair. The woman had no idea how heavy she was, but she knew her mother-in-law could not walk due to obesity. The daughter-in-law did not know the real reason her mother-in-law was in a wheelchair. The house she lived in was a total mess with many people living there, and her father-in-law had lung cancer and still smoked cigarettes all the time. The daughter-in-law said she and her husband, the woman's son, were so embarrassed that they let the situation with his mother, Maureen, get this out of hand. Her embarrassment even on the phone telling me all this was just so overwhelming. I could hear the tears in her voice. She and her husband couldn't stand visiting his mother anymore. It was just too tragic and painful. Was I willing to go there to her home and see if I could help? She told me it would be very difficult. I had no idea how difficult.

I told her I was always willing to try and couldn't imagine a situation I couldn't tolerate. I had grown up in a smoker's house with alcoholism, so how much worse could this house be?

Maureen was well over three hundred fifty pounds and lived mostly in her living room, where she watched game shows with the volume on the TV turned way up. The house was a total mess. It was about 1,500 square feet with six to eight relatives living there with her at all times with most rooms made into bedrooms filled with laundry. Everyone in the house was severely obese except her husband. Her husband was rail thin from his lung cancer. He stayed in the garage, chain-smoking cigarettes and never once said hi to me. No one was happy I was there, including Maureen, the mother-in-law in the wheelchair I was supposed to be helping.

Her son, who was also over three hundred pounds and about thirty years old, would try to make trouble when I was there. He would eat a whole pizza in front of us, kind of like a big Fuck You, and blasted the TV so I could barely talk to his mother. In the second week, I lost my cool. I told the family, "Enough. You want to watch your mother die in a wheelchair and recliner from obesity while you live financially off of her, great. I can't. I am here to help her, and I want all of you out of here while I am here. Otherwise, I leave and never come back." I was trembling with anger and the emotion that people were killing themselves from obesity.

The family agreed not to be in the house when I was there to work with their mother Maureen. When I first started with her, she couldn't even stand up on her own. She would do this severe rocking movement to get her body weight behind her and propel herself forward as a family member grabbed her arms, pulled her up out of the recliner, then helped her to her wheelchair or walker. This happened every time if she had to go to the bathroom or to get something. She was only sixty-three years old and recently retired from her job. Someone had to be home with her all the time just to get her out of a chair.

I really liked this client. I liked her personality. Maureen wasn't dumb or naïve. She knew what a mess she had done to her body and how sick her whole family was physically and mentally. She confided in me she had no idea how to fix the situation or how her home life had gotten so out of control. She was very sad that her son and his wife couldn't even stand to visit her anymore. Maureen missed them and cried about how she had become an embarrassment to them. Family meant everything to her. I showed Maureen her family could be her reason to lose weight. I convinced her that we would make progress quickly, and she could show her son how wonderfully she was doing with her weight and getting more mobile. Her son and his wife would be proud of her and want to see her again. She looked at me with these eyes of hope. I knew I could help her if she just believed in me.

Within a month, I could get her to get herself up out of her recliner without help, get her to stand with a walker, and not use anyone to help her go to the bathroom or kitchen. She was so very proud of her hard work and smiled through the exertion of her exercises. She reduced her junk food intake and was drinking more water and not just sodas. When her family brought in junk food, Maureen tried very hard not to eat it. I told her, "This is about you, not your family or anyone else, just be strong for you." "You have come so far, don't stop" was my constant mantra to her. She began to smile more and would be happy when I came over to work with her.

Now for the graphic reality check. I want non-obese people to understand the difficulty obese people have every day. She was so obese she couldn't dress herself. Her husband dressed her every day. She used massive amounts of talcum powder to control the sweating under her large folds of skin. If she didn't use the talcum powder, the sweat would cause bacteria to form and large rashes to take over her body. When she used the bathroom, someone else had to wipe her crotch for her because she couldn't reach her crotch with her own arms after urination or defecation.

She had pus oozing out of her legs all the time. Yellow thick puss came out of her pores. She had compression wraps to put on her legs that had to be washed and rewrapped on her legs daily by her daughter. These wraps were specially ordered for her from her doctors at Kaiser Permanente, her insurance provider.

Maureen was so obese; she could not sleep lying down because the weight of her breasts and excess fat on her chest pressed on her lungs. She slept in an oversized recliner in the living room, halfway sitting up. Her spine was massively crooked from sitting all the time in her recliner and all that weight bearing down on her. Her height had reduced by five inches from the way she hunched over. Her spine was now an S shape with one hip about four inches higher than the other one. I knew that even if I could get her moving, this back and hip malformation would never be fixed and would cause her a lifetime of pain.

I had the family buy her an adjustable bed with a pulley system installed above it in the bedroom, so she could get in and out of it independently. It took her one month of hard work to get in and out of bed by herself using the pully system. She slowly learned how to manipulate her body, but her legs had become so large she was unable to move them without the use of her arms.

Maureen was thrilled to sleep in bed with her husband for the first time in ten years. She and her husband slept together for three months before he passed away from his lung cancer. He still never once looked at me or said a word to me in all the hours I worked with his wife.

After her husband passed away, she swallowed her grief and kept working hard to get physically better. I think she only took one day off from working out with me to go to the funeral. Friends of hers came over and marveled at her weight loss and her ability to walk around the house. Maureen could answer the front door when someone came over and could feed her own dogs. Her son and daughter-in-law came over every Sunday and marveled at her weight loss and mobility. They were eternally grateful to me for being willing to help her. Her friends took her to the bingo hall to play and socialize. Maureen was blossoming as a human being. I was so proud of her. Seeing her three times a week was delightful. She wasn't just my client; she was my friend.

One Monday, when I got to her house for her workout, she told me she had something to tell me, something serious. "Vanessa, I am bleeding." She didn't know if it was her bladder, vagina, or anus, just that when she went to the bathroom, there was massive amounts of blood sometimes. "Like something broke" was how she described it to me. She now took care of herself in the bathroom and could shower on her own. She had lost about forty pounds; this is an estimation. I never got her on a scale, but she was remarkably smaller and very mobile.

When people get this obese, they can no longer leave their homes, and their doctors take care of their health needs, prescriptions, and mental health services, over the phone or by email. She took over ten pills a day for diabetes, pain, depression, and cholesterol—all delivered by mail to her home.

I asked her, "When is the last time you saw a gynecologist?" She couldn't remember but felt it had been at least seven years since she had been in to see a doctor in person. She couldn't go to the gynecologist because she had become too heavy to put her feet up in the stirrups. When she lay down on an examination table, the weight of her chest crushed her, making breathing impossible, so she panicked.

I called one of her girlfriends who agreed to take her to the doctor, and we made the appointment. I knew the doctor well; he had helped one of my other obese patients. He had been so happy I was working with and helping Maureen. He told Maureen how lucky she was to get to work with me. I had great success with other patients of his, and he always recommended me. I didn't feel lucky to work with her. This time I knew something was seriously wrong that was out of my control.

I was with another client when my phone rang. I usually don't answer the phone when I am with a client but knew this was the doctor's office. He told me Maureen had stage four ovarian cancer. Because she was still obese at three hundred twenty pounds, no anesthesiologist would help with the surgery. He told me what I already knew. If Maureen hadn't had been this obese, she would have seen a doctor every couple of years, and they could have caught the cancer sooner. He was sorry. I thanked the doctor for telling me and hung up the phone. I didn't know what to do. I knew I had to be strong and keep showing up for her.

I continued to see her three times a week. My client was now on painkillers and would fall asleep during our workouts. Maureen passed away peacefully within two months. I was devastated. She had worked so hard, had found some freedom and happiness with weight loss, and still her obesity killed her. After she died, for over two years I stopped taking people over three hundred pounds. I couldn't take it emotionally. I just couldn't have another one die on me. I was taking it all very personally.

My first personal training job was also an obese woman. I had just left a corporate job I hated, my divorce was final, and I was on the verge of bankruptcy with my mortgage payments three months behind. I was lost and had no clue what to do in my life. A friend of mine asked me, "Vanessa, will you help my sister lose some weight? She got really heavy after college."

At this time, I was teaching a little tennis, but I had never considered becoming a personal trainer. I hated gyms and felt most personal trainers had no clue what they were doing with clients, let alone their own bodies. Some personal trainers were bodybuilders on steroids, some were just pretty girls in small clothes, and some personal trainers were even overweight and out of shape themselves. Also, I didn't want to work for so little money; I needed to find a "real job." I had never met a personal trainer who made a living working in a gym.

"Vanessa, you are the fittest person I know and, well, you don't have a job now, so what do you have to lose? Take her to the park, jump around with her—you know that jumping on a bench thing you do—run around, do some push-ups, whatever—just help her. I will give you one hundred dollars a week, then at least you can afford to feed your dogs," my friend said.

I was very angry at my friend. I don't like charity and had never helped anyone lose weight. I had helped people fix weak joints, crooked backs, and put on muscle definition but not in any official capacity—and definitely not for money. The more I thought about it, the more I wanted to give it a try. If I had lost sixty pounds in a summer as a teenager, maybe I could do this, and my friend was right. I needed to feed the dogs.

My friend's sister, Marybeth, walked up to meet me at a local park, and my first impression was that she was exceptionally beautiful. Long flowing blond hair, beautiful teeth, and about one hundred pounds overweight. My friend had said his sister put on weight, but I had no idea how much weight.

She introduced herself, and I asked a few questions. Marybeth was not taking any prescription medications. She was twenty-five years old and not fond of sweating or traditional sports. She blamed the weight on having a desk job and was in complete denial about how heavy she had become in the past two years.

I never asked how much she weighed. She wore stretch clothes all the time. We worked out for about an hour. Marybeth broke a sweat, ran a little, did some arm workouts, I made her laugh. I never asked her to do something she couldn't do physically. I told her I would be at the park Monday to Friday at 7:00 a.m., and she could join me or not; it was her decision. Her brother was paying me either way. Marybeth could stop working out with me at any time. I told her I just wanted to help her until I found a real job.

She showed up the next day and the next and the next. Twice in the first month, she cussed me out. Complete screaming and yelling at me in public. I was patient. I don't think I had ever been patient with anyone with two legs in my life. If you were a dog or a horse, great, but a human? No, I never had patience for a human before—no wonder my marriages failed. I knew I cared about her and wanted her to lose the weight, and l let her scream her frustration at me. I just hoped Marybeth would keep showing up and working out with me.

She kept showing up to work out and apologized for her behavior many times. I shrugged it off because I understood her frustration with her body. Soon, Marybeth had to pull up her stretch pants, loose from weight loss, between exercises. I got to the park late one morning and an attractive man was talking to her. She beamed and smiled from his attention. She was down by my estimate about forty pounds.

She got promoted at work and wanted to pay me more. I declined. Her brother and I had a deal. It took two years. Marybeth lost one hundred and five pounds. She has kept the weight off for over six years now.

Marybeth moved away, got married, and now has a beautiful family. I don't get to see Marybeth often, but she calls me her angel. I call her my start. She made me realize I could do this, and whatever this was, it was becoming my career.

# CHAPTER 13

# WORKOUTS AND LIFESTYLE CHANGES FOR OVERWEIGHT/ OBESE CLIENTS

I never ask a client to do anything they physically can't. Ever. Asking a one hundred-pound overweight woman to get on the floor and do abdominal exercises is a recipe for disaster. They can't get down to the floor and back up on their own. It is humiliating for them, unproductive and painful. Don't ever humiliate another human being if you are trying to help them. No good comes of it.

First, I find out how much a client's body hurts. Knees, hips, shoulders, backs are common problem areas. I find out about their daily lives, how they get around, how much they sleep. I don't approach food at all for probably the first three weeks. Overweight people have been hearing for years, if not their whole lives, they eat the wrong things and too much. They don't need to hear criticism right off the bat.

I avoid criticism always.

Instead, I focus on positive movement. Movement that will raise their heart rates slightly and work up a little sweat. I make all of my clients wear heart rate monitoring watches, so I can keep track of their efforts. I try to make the workouts fun and point out how moving more will help them feel better physically and mentally. Workouts with me are an ever-changing rotation of body movements to hit different muscles and body parts.

Learning how to get off a chair without using their arms, walking with proper posture, improving overall flexibility—all are great starting points for obese people. I want to help them live life more pain-free. Sometimes we may do an exercise for just ten seconds, sometimes for two minutes, depending on the cardiovascular and respiratory condition of the client.

We always finish on a happy note of accomplishment. And drink lots of water. I always remind them to drink lots of water when they leave.

Water issues are interesting. When I first started working as a personal trainer and needed clients, I would put up with

"I hate water and won't drink it." I would let this negative attitude toward water go and would try to just encourage the obese client in other ways. Not anymore. Now if an obese client says they won't even drink water, that is a stopping point for me. I need the client to be at least willing to drink water, or they won't do anything else I ask.

As I write this book, I can remember five clients I have parted ways with over their not even being willing to drink water at all.

Here is one.

Mary's son was getting married in six months. She wanted to slim down to look better in the wedding pictures. Mary kept telling me how healthy she was, and she didn't have any medical or physical problems. In my opinion, she was at least sixty pounds overweight, and she was lying to me and herself, but I kept quiet. She took four prescription pills a day, but all of her friends did, she said, and Mary just wanted me to work her out so she could get a waist back. She had that hard belly fat we used to see only on men but has become common on women now too. Her back was very swayed from the weight of her stomach. I tried to tell her weight loss didn't work that way. We couldn't make her body just lose weight in one section. She didn't want to hear it.

"How much water do you drink a day?" I asked.

"Oh, I hate water; don't make me drink water. I just won't drink water," she responded.

"Won't" is a strong response. I told Mary if she wouldn't even drink water, she would never lose the weight.

"Losing weight is not just about moving your body but also about what goes into your body."

She lasted as a client for one month and never lost any weight. In fact, she is the only client I have ever had who, after a month, actually gained weight while working with me.

No one gets to be sixty, eighty, or one hundred pounds over-weight overnight. Lifestyle changes don't happen overnight either. Coming to see me is a first step, and I slowly bring in lifestyle changes that will fit my clients' lives and help them live happier, pain-free lives.

Water is the first step. I know this sounds repetitive, but ideally, I want the client to be drinking thirty ounces of water first thing in the morning then again around 3:00 p.m. for a minimum of sixty ounces of water a day regardless of anything else they drink during the day. It may take a client three to four months just for this water drinking to be a habit.

I want them learning to move more every day, not just when they come to see me for their workouts. Garmin or Apple watches can monitor their movements and keep track of their step counts every day. Step counts can be great motivators. I encourage them to do small things every day to get more steps in. Park at the end of a parking lot when going to the grocery store. Go outside into the backyard and just walk around. Get out in the sun and take in some Vitamin D every day.

I had a client who came to me because her boyfriend, a large Silicon Valley company CEO, knew of me and suggested it. Sybil wasn't really into seeing a personal trainer. She had a hurting back, very swayed, and a belly that stuck out over a foot from her body over her feet. She was only carrying extra fat around her mid-section, and because her back hurt, she would lace her fingers under her belly and hold her belly up to try to ease the pain of her back when she stood or walked. Sybil was only forty years old, and with that large belly and the way she held it with her hands, it made her look eight months pregnant. People asked her all the time when the baby was due.

Sybil was the CEO's administrative assistant when they first met. He started dating her when his first marriage was breaking up. He would tell me how nice Sybil was to him when he was in mental pain over his marriage ending. He spoke of her kindness fondly.

For her, he was an amazing catch, and she knew it. A wealthy CEO, he paid for her apartment, and now was paying for her personal trainer. Sybil didn't go to business dinners with him or out in public with him. She was too embarrassed about being fat, about being in pain with her bad back. She didn't feel accomplished at work and didn't speak intelligently enough around "those people." Sybil said she was fine only seeing her boyfriend in private because he was so good and nice to her. She was worried if she didn't fix her back, so she could have more sex with him, he would dump her. I'll be honest, I wasn't fine with any of this and wanted her to get some self-respect. I know I said that to her too much and tried to contain my personal beliefs and just work her out and help her with her food choices.

The boyfriend CEO paid for two sessions per week. Sybil usually only came to one session a week. Twenty minutes before the second session, she would tell me her back hurt too much for her to work out, or she was too tired from work to come in. She would beg me not to tell her boyfriend she had skipped a session because he was so proud of her for trying to get fit. I told her I didn't work that way. He was paying for the sessions. I would have to tell him he was paying for sessions she didn't attend.

He bought her an Apple watch in the beginning like I asked him to, so I could monitor her step count and heart rate. Many days, she came in for her workout and had barely walked two thousand steps in the whole day. Sybil didn't care about her lack of movement. She wasn't willing to put in any effort to change her body. She said she was in too much pain and couldn't walk even though her doctor said he could find nothing wrong with her back. Sybil had been to at least five doctors who told her nothing was wrong with her back and they didn't know why she was in such pain. I knew it was because her belly was so large, making her back sway. I finally had to be rough with her after about four weeks into those half-ass workouts. Honestly, I was sick of her excuses and her not even being willing to try to move her body.

Sybil hadn't lost any weight in the four weeks. We were getting nowhere except she was satisfying the boyfriend by coming to me and telling him she was trying to move and workout. I told her it wasn't working out. She was unwilling or unable to put any effort into cutting down her food intake or exercising more or drinking water. I felt I was wasting her boyfriend's money. Sybil left my studio in a huff. It was a bad breakup between us, and I felt I was unprofessional.

I called the boyfriend CEO and told him I thought his girlfriend, Sybil, might be better with another personal trainer. I was unable to help her with her back pain or any weight loss. He said he understood and told me he wanted to pay me for her booked sessions through the end of the month. I thanked him, and he said, "I was going to break up with her anyway, she is not my type. I just was nice to her because she was nice to me when I needed her, and I couldn't take her in public anyway. Thanks for trying, Vanessa; I appreciate all your efforts and honesty. Hey, anyway, I was talking about you to a mutual acquaintance, and well, he thought we had a lot in common. Would you like to attend a business dinner with me next week? I think we would have fun together, and well, you will know other people there." As desperate as I was for a date, I wasn't *that* desperate. I declined.

This wasn't in the personal training manual. In fact, all of this personal stuff wasn't ever discussed in any trainings I had been to. I have now learned that the mental aspect of helping people fix their bodies is even more important than what I have them do physically. And the best way to be a good personal trainer is to practice patience and silence.

So, in review, I get obese clients moving. Moving gently so they can learn to use their bodies again. I get them to drink water daily and move their bodies daily. I structure workouts so their daily lives will be easier. I try to instill in them constant movement and paying attention to what they eat.

Realize change is hard and be patient with yourself if you are obese. Take the time to get to where you want to be and just be happy you are making progress. Everyone goes backward sometimes. Shake it off and just walk a few minutes when you feel sad. The blood circulating always makes you feel better, and then you are moving forward.

# CHAPTER 14

# DAD BODS AND THE CONSTANTLY SITTING MAN

L ife has changed drastically for humans in the United States in the last fifty years. Now, most people, especially college-educated upper-middle-class people and above, work a job where they sit at their desks and type all day on their computers or talk on the phone. It's very interesting to see how the bodies of these men all look similar when they get to their fifties and early sixties. They have hard belly fat, a flat butt (which should be muscular), their necks stick out four to six inches in front of their shoulders, they arch their lower backs all the time to compensate for their large bellies, and they walk with their feet out in front of them like a duck. Some men are severely crooked with a shoulder three to four inches higher on one side, depending how they lean on their desks.

Most men started to go to the doctor for the first time in their forties. They have a low testosterone level, feel sluggish and stressed, and have high blood pressure and high cholesterol. Then their doctors begin their prescription drug therapies.

Doctors give out drugs to save lives. Drugs can make our symptoms recede relatively quickly; but in the long term, how these men got these unhealthy issues remain, and the men usually still don't feel happy in their bodies. These men decide to try diets and exercises but get hurt quickly by trying to be the athletes they were in high school and fail to get the weight off, so they give up. Most have been gaining weight over the course of a couple of decades and have become very resigned to just being heavier in their midlives than they were in their twenties. Because as an American society, seventy-five percent of the population is overweight, acceptance sets in with these men. All their friends have "dad bodies" and take prescription drugs, so they just go with it.

Injuries, from strain or immobility, begin to affect everyday life for men over forty. These men start with sore shoulders, necks, backs, and knees, and the litany of pain issues gets longer the more sessions they attend. Here are the common issues:

- Eat processed food
- Eat out more than five times a week

- Drink too much alcohol
- Smoke cigars and/or cigarettes
- Don't exercise regularly
- Take so many prescription drugs, their kidneys hurt
- Don't drink water
- Don't sleep enough, or well
- Are exhausted
- Have impotence issues
- Are depressed or anxious in their home or work life
- Have frequent headaches
- Have overall body pains

Let's meet some of these men and see how their lives have changed after working out with me.

Albert said he had tried five personal trainers in the past few weeks and hadn't settled on one to work with yet and wanted to try me also. Would I be available to come up to his home some morning this week? He had a gym set up in his home. I made a time, got his address, and didn't think much of it. I didn't google his name; this was just another personal training appointment for me.

The home was amazing on a few acres, and beautiful. His impressive gym had a weight machine, treadmill, bike, mirrors, stacks of free weights—all the regular stuff you would have if you copied a gym out of a magazine. The man was in his mid-sixties, slightly overweight, and looked like he had been a smoker. His body was crooked.

"So, what do you do for fun and how can I help you?" I asked.

He told me he had recently retired from a CEO position and now was sitting on many company boards, so his days were full. He golfed regularly.

"How do you golf with that right shoulder so low and the sway in your back?" I asked honestly. I didn't wait for a reply. "I can fix that," I told him.

He smiled. "Can you see me three times a week?" he asked.

I was in. Albert had very little balance and was crooked and needed to lose a few pounds. He was also more than willing to do the work to make his body straighter and healthier to enjoy life. But he was so impatient!!! If Albert couldn't do a simple exercise easily, he wanted to speed through and do it halfway and give up. I would laugh when he expected his body to be better.

"Why would you expect it to be better when you haven't worked at it. Is that how the companies you work with succeed, through neglect and bad treatment?" I asked often.

After about five years together, he stopped by my studio mid-day to ask me a question. I was working with two women who were shocked at how young and fit he looked for his age. They thought he had great square shoulders. I laughed. I have a thing for shoulders, men's and women's. He had been working out with me for many years very successfully.

Everyone has those "Ah, ha!" moments, and here was his. He went to Hong Kong for business and always had custom dress shirts made there. The tailor was impressed with his smaller neck, smaller waist, and good shoulders. He had to call me from Hong Kong to tell me how happy he was in his new clothes. His wife laughed. "Sorry Vanessa, he just had to tell you," she told me. I didn't mind; it made me smile.

He lives for his grandkids. They are the light of his life. "Vanessa, yesterday my grandson ran at me and jumped in my arms, and I could hold him! My back didn't even hurt!" He worked out to be fit enough to play with his grandkids physically and watch them grow up. He still lives life to the fullest, finding balance with his food and alcohol consumption. Even on the days I don't work out with him, he goes into his gym to do some light weights and stretching—wonderful life changes to keep him happy and healthy.

I worked with a CEO that disliked overweight people in his personal and professional life. If he hired you to work at his company and you were upper management, meaning you had to fly for work, he would not pay for an upgraded seat. (Obese people can't fit comfortably in coach seats.) When he hired you, he would say that you had three months to lose the weight to fit into a regular airline seat. For those three months of your probation, he would pay for a personal trainer to help you. I had been instructed to work with three new hires. Only one succeeded. Here he is.

## OUR FIRST MEETING

The new employee, Charlie, didn't even look at me at our first meeting. Charlie's anger at having to work out, especially with me, a woman, was apparent. I tried to have a conversation; Charlie wasn't having it.

"What did you have for dinner last night?" I asked him after analyzing his body and guessing he was over sixty pounds overweight.

He proudly stated, "A baked potato with sour cream, a steak, and three scotches."

"Great," I replied, "you can only have two of the three for dinner tonight, that is too many calories."

"Fine, I will give up the potato," he replied very sarcastically.

"I am cool with that" was my answer as he huffed in disbelief as he turned his back on me and continued with whatever exercise I was having him do.

Charlie hated working out and especially hated the sweating of alcohol out of his pores. He hated even more that he could barely do any exercise for more than one minute without needing a rest to try to breathe. Breathing was almost impossible for him because his heart rate would become so high. Charlie was seething his anger on me, and I just laughed it off every time, upsetting him even more. He thought I was laughing at him because he was fat and someone else was paying for me. That wasn't it at all. I was laughing at his defiance and recognizing that same character flaw in myself, defiance. I knew I had to break through his defiance if we were going to succeed so he could keep his job.

After his first week, I wore him out mentally. I stayed overly upbeat. Then he got honest and looked at me with very pained eyes, saying, "Vanessa, this is the best job I have ever had, and I can't lose it. I am sixty-two years old. No one else is going to hire me at this level at this age. I can't get fired from this job." The tears were ready to fall out of his eyes. I felt his emotional pain welling up and so near the surface. He looked like he might explode.

"I know that," I said. "And your boss is paying for a private personal trainer, his own personal trainer. Don't you think you should take that gift for all it is worth? Would getting healthy really be that horrible, or would you rather die broke and fat?"

I knew this was a rough thing to say. This is a truth that I accepted in my own life. I knew this was hard for Charlie to hear. I was getting weary of people who just accepted their weight-induced limited mobility. I told him I understood the pain of being overweight and truly believed he would love the new body I could help him achieve—if he would just accept my help.

I was ready for him to just quit and walk out the door. Charlie's face was red with anger and humiliation.

Instead, Charlie turned to me and with tears in his eyes said, "I always fail at losing weight. I am sorry, Vanessa. I am not angry at you. I am disgusted with myself and my lack of willpower."

My response: "Bummer, let's go for a jog."

See, I couldn't handle the pain I saw in him. The pain I had felt as an overweight unathletic child, the pain I saw in many clients who feel they will always be overweight, out of shape and unable to change. We walked/jogged for over thirty minutes, and by the end of this run, he was laughing at my stupid jokes. Charlie agreed to give my methods an honest try this time and stop being rude to me.

Charlie needed more help than most clients because his whole life needed to change in ten weeks so he could keep his job.

I hired him a personal chef to prepare him and his wife three meals a week and leave instructions for heating the prepared meals. Charlie and his wife learned to eat better. He recognized he was using food as a crutch to get through the hard aspects of his life. Please note I didn't tell him this. He came to this realization on his own. He never knew if he was hungry, a common issue for my clients. Most people just eat food because it is time, dinner time, lunchtime, etc. He learned drinking alcohol the night before seeing me was just torture. Yeah, I work out hung-over people extra hard instead of saying anything about their drinking of alcohol. He cut back on drinking the nights before seeing me, which became a habit of drinking less overall.

Charlie recognized he used food and alcohol as crutches to drown the unhappiness of life. He asked me if all clients did this with food and alcohol. I told him I couldn't speak for all of my clients, but I knew at many times in my life I did the same and still do occasionally. We are human, we hurt, and we can only do our best to fix ourselves.

At the end of the three months, he had lost forty pounds and kept his job. He ran his first 5K with me at the end of four months. Charlie has excelled at his job and looks great, smiling and laughing all the time. He brought his wife in to meet me one day. She thanked me for helping her husband and bringing back the man she had married and loved so much. She looked at Charlie with such love I was beyond jealous but at the same time thankful I could help. They left arm in arm. She kissed his cheek as they walked out the door. I continue to see him two times a week four years later, but ha, now he has to pay for his own personal training!

I received an email from a website referral. David told me he was overweight and had knee issues. I have recently lost three over-weight women who died from their obesity and wasn't anxious to take on another client over three hundred pounds. The pain of those three dying female clients was just too fresh in my mind. The man had to go on a business trip and couldn't start working out with me for three weeks. I usually just ignore client's phone calls like this. I tell them to call me when they are ready. If a client doesn't start within four to five days of that first phone call, they rarely start with me ever. They lose momentum.

David was different, though. He set his appointment for three weeks out and showed up. The man looked at me kind of sideways on our first meeting. David had lost the weight many times, but he always gained it back, and then some. He seemed sad to me, though I knew he had been successful with his career. His weight was holding him back not just physically but mentally. He was slightly angry at life in general. I made him get on the scale at the first meeting, something I had never done before with a client. I just couldn't chance it. *Cool, two hundred and ninety-six pounds. I could do this* was my thought, and I smiled. (I didn't tell him about my over-three-hundred-pound-everyone-dies-on-me thing for a few months.)

David's weight loss had been slow and consistent, sometimes backwards. He had knee issues due to the pounds he had been carrying. Running was difficult for him, but he hiked every weekend for six miles or so. He completed two 5Ks and one five-mile race, placing right in the middle for his age group. He was thrilled to exercise with others.

He had hard belly fat, and I warned him how strange his body would look when this fat began to come off. This fat starts to soften around the groin area first, sitting wiggly under the hard belly. Clients look uncomfortable at this stage of weight loss, but it lets me know the body is responding to less food and more exercise. Our human bodies want to be efficient. Food cravings are a problem he will have to confront all of his life. Bread is his downfall, and David just can't help but keep it in his house no matter how many times I tell him to just not buy it.

Food is so personal with clients. Food is not just nourishment for our bodies; it is our comfort and security for our brains.

David has been with me for over five years. He lost sixty pounds while working with me and kept the weight off. He still works at it and has about forty more pounds to go. David won't give up. I won't let him.

An executive assistant called me about her boss, Nathan, who wanted to get fit in two months. He wanted to be fit so he could take his kids skiing. The previous year he had blown his knee on the ski mountain. Nathan felt this accident happened because he wasn't "ski conditioned." The executive assistant thought he had about thirty pounds to lose. I didn't respond to this statement. I knew getting "ski conditioned" wasn't possible without even seeing the man but agreed to take Nathan on as a client.

Nathan wanted to work out three evenings a week and book them solidly right away. I don't normally work this way. I want a client to do their first hour with me and then decide if this is the right decision for them. I want a first appointment to see if I am the right fit for their fitness journey. Then we can decide together how many days to do a week depending on their physical capabilities, finances, and time constraints.

I have now learned that evening appointments rarely work for anyone. Could be me or the client or both, we just fail together. Past 7:30 p.m., it is just too difficult. People want to be home and are exhausted from their workdays.

Nathan came in for the first time well over sixty pounds over-weight and very unhealthy looking. Kind of a light grey skin color and a cold clammy sweat even before starting to work out. His breathing was more of a wheeze and he said he did not have asthma. I guessed he had high blood pressure also. He did not think he was unhealthy enough to need regular doc-tor visits and had not had a blood test or full physical ever. He was thirty-nine years old. He refused to go see a doctor when I asked him to. He also refused to use the blood pressure cuff I keep in the studio.

Nathan was a high-level engineer. He boasted about how much money he made at the company he worked for, how every company in town wanted him. He told me how great of a gamer he was (on the weekends, he would sit on the couch and game for eight to ten hours at a time, believing it healthier than outdoor sports) and that he really wasn't that unhealthy. He just never really wanted to be thinner, but his wife kept nagging him. Nathan talked down to me as if I was stupid. I let it go.

We did two weeks together. I don't know who hated the work-outs more, him or me. He detested everything we did and really didn't want to be there. He would not do an exercise for more than fifteen seconds without being out of breath. After two weeks I wished him well, but I didn't think we were a fit and he should try to find someone else to help him. He didn't care. He told me I was stupid to give up his money.

A fifty-one-year-old high-level successful tech manager who had left his job recently called me. He now was going to look at consulting or working at a startup and had a few months between jobs. Joe was not too overweight, maybe thirty pounds, but had a resting heart rate of eighty and knew he wasn't healthy. He was also carrying all of his fat as hard belly fat.

Boy, was he stiff! Neck stuck forward from working at a computer all the time, large hard stomach fat (which always worries me), hamstrings and hips a mess! Just so tight! Tight hamstrings make the lower back hurt all the time.

Joe had a super willing attitude from the beginning. He has been with me for about four years, always willing to try any exercise. The weight is off, he looks great, ran his first half- marathon, and continues to run with his wife and daughter with the whole family embracing exercise and healthy eating. I always have to convince him to stretch and ice when he is not with me. Some things just don't become a habit easily.

His arms look incredible, and we are very close to that six-pack look his wife wants!

Richard called me and bitched me out about my Google ranking: it wasn't high enough. He couldn't find me the first time he searched for a personal trainer, and that upset him. (If you don't know, Google rankings, like the first listing for "San Jose personal trainer," will cost you over fifteen dollars a click or about one thousand dollars a month). He wanted to meet me first in person before booking a workout with me, which was fine.

Richard came at the end of the day as I was cleaning up. This professionally dressed sixty-year-old man, about thirty pounds overweight, had arthritis starting in his knees and shoulders. He had seen doctors for the arthritis pain and wanted quick fixes. He was begging his doctors for surgery as quickly as possible. I work with many people with arthritis, and if I can get them moving every day, the arthritis will be tolerable or completely go away depending on the severity. With arthritis, it is all about keeping the inflammation down in the body.

I agreed to see Richard twice a week. I immediately didn't like him. He was very passive-aggressive and kept going on about how great his other personal trainer was, an ex-circus performer. He enjoyed a lifestyle I didn't agree with, so I asked him not to talk about certain aspects during our workouts. This was the first time I had ever had to set those boundaries. We mutually disliked each other.

He respected me as a personal trainer, though, and agreed to try "this exercise thing" for a year before seeking surgeries. He improved remarkably in three months and, within a year, felt mostly free of pain. His knees no longer hurt, he was able to run a little, he lost over twenty pounds, and he stopped looking for doctors to give him a quick fix. Richard left me remarkably better, and we had become friends. He had to move away. I hope he is still doing well.

These men were all remarkably similar: overweight, stiff, and neglectful of their bodies, hurting them in their careers and family lives. Now let's see how to help them get a body they will love and use.

# CHAPTER 15

# WORKOUTS AND LIFESTYLE CHANGES FOR MIDDLE-AGED MEN

Whether I'm with a first-time or long-term client, most of my workouts begin with a warm-up, so I can analyze each client's abilities. During the warm-up, we get the hips and back moving, and I look for imbalances, assess their posture, and consider weight differences or new pain areas. A slight heart rate rise to about one hundred beats per minute in this warm-up phase would be normal. New middle-aged clients develop a redness or flushed look around their necks, a sign of high blood pressure. Men also try to push themselves harder, trying to prove something, so I bring them back in the beginning to understanding a slow warm-up before we work out. I check their mental health. I tell a few jokes, ask about the family, their jobs. The trick here is to relax and destress them as the workout begins. I also want them to learn to feel their bodies and especially the blood pressure issues.

Twelve to fifteen minutes of cardio follows. I like to mix up my cardio: the rowing machine one day, the stair machine the next, or stationary bike or treadmill. We could do some ladder work or other bodyweight exercise. I am big on jumping, so good for the bones and involves many muscles and body parts. I stay with the client during this, talking to them, monitoring their form and heart rate. They may need to slow down, speed up, or take a few minor rests to get to the desired twelve to fifteen minutes. I am always shooting for a heart rate over one hundred fifty-five for at least seven to eight minutes but not over one hundred sixty-five. Over one hundred sixty-five beats per minute is a danger zone and makes the client uncomfortable. Cardio should always feel like work but not like hell. This cardio is important to build the heart and lungs. Breathing has to go with heartbeat, or side stitches or nausea develop. Breathing during exercise is something to be practiced and doesn't come easily.

Next comes some weight workouts, alternating between arms or legs, depending on the day, for about ten to fifteen minutes. Men want muscle definition more than women, and we work toward getting definition especially in the arms after a solid year together. Getting muscle definition involves serious work, pain, and exertion, not just from the muscle groups but from the heart too. That is why we hear of professional bodybuilders dying from heart attacks. To get definition, we actually have to rip and build up the desired muscle. If this is what my client is looking for, he should understand that we can't even work on this for probably a year. First, we get body fat down, then endurance, then strength, then definition.

If the client is fit enough to get on the floor comfortably and get off the floor by themselves, we will go down and do mat work. Please note, I don't ask clients to make themselves embarrassed by being too heavy, having too bad of knees or hips, or having blood pressure issues that will make mat work uncomfortable. We can do some work off a bench or box, if that is easier for the client, so we can work out the back and core.

I have never met a client that didn't want a toner midsection. I try to spend twenty minutes doing mat work: stretching, core work, flexibility, and arm strength exercises. During mat work, I try to get them to talk about incorporating exercise, moving, and good eating into their daily lifestyle. No one gets fit working out with me just once or twice a week. I encourage my clients to change their lifestyle and perform an exercise they enjoy every day.

Men in this age group now realize the damage they have done to their bodies; being overweight, having poor nutrition, avoiding exercise, and sitting at desk jobs have caused mental and physical stress. They realize they are no longer young and are desperate to feel like their twenty-year-old self again.

Drinking enough water, at least sixty ounces broken into thirty ounces in the morning first thing and thirty ounces again at 3:00 p.m. is a great start. Avoiding the snacking at your desk and keeping the alcohol to a maximum of two drinks a day.

Discussions of alcohol can be tricky. I just try to keep it to the facts and at the same time make it personal about myself and not condescending to the client. "You know if I drink two glasses of wine the night before I run, then my heart rate is up ten beats a minute the next day." I don't make a condemnation of the client's own drinking. I try to show them how their drinking affects their everyday life and maybe they should take a look at how much alcohol they drink.

Staying up late at night is a killer. We all have trouble sleeping as we get older, so try to get to bed and shoot for eight hours of sleep. Pay attention to your body clock. If you always seem to wake up at 6:00 a.m. without an alarm, then you would have to get to bed by 9:45 p.m., then be asleep by 10:00 p.m. to get eight hours of sleep. Learn to listen to your body. If you feel tired, there is a reason. Nap if you can, depending on your work and life schedule. Good sleep and rest are just as important to overall health as working out and nutrition.

I try to get the men I work with to involve their families in good eating habits and exercise regimes. If you take long runs on the weekends, have your kids ride their bikes along with you, so they can hold your water and encourage you. Make them part of helping you get fit and healthy. Take family hikes together.

Go to the park and play Frisbee or football or basketball, even if you can barely play. Then you are teaching them to exercise and have fun with other people. Involve the whole family in shopping at farmer's markets and cooking so good food habits are passed around the family and encouraged.

Practice deep breathing and slowing down your brain for two to five minutes a day. I don't call it meditation unless the client is open to meditation or interested in the benefits of meditation. I want them to learn to use their full lung capacity to exercise better and release stress.

Learn to love their bodies and not be condescending of their physical condition. Men lose weight faster than women, and even at middle age they can spiral that football, hit that golf ball three hundred yards, run their first marathon, bench two hundred pounds, all those physical things they wanted to do in their younger days and gave up when life took over.

We work toward the goals that make them happy.

Okay, I do have a personal thing. Shoulders. I always try to put square shoulders on a man through weight work. It's a great look in a t-shirt or business suit. I think you could identify a client of mine, male or female, because I always put pretty shoulders on them.

# CHAPTER 16

# WOMEN 40-70 CAN STILL LOOK HOT AND BE INCREDIBLE!

n 1972, Title IX passed. This landmark legislation changed sports for women. Without Title IX, I wouldn't be a personal trainer and runner today, and we definitely wouldn't have so many women with college degrees.

The following is the original text as written and signed into law by President Richard Nixon in 1972:

*No person in the United States shall, based on sex, be excluded from participation in, be denied the benefits of, or be subjected to*

*discrimination under any education program or activity receiving*
*Federal financial assistance.*

—Cornell Law School's Legal Information
Institute (20 U.S. Code § 1681—Sex)

Basically, this law meant that women were entitled to college scholarships for sports and athletic ability just like men.

In the 1970s, I believed this would be the heart of the women's movement, where women would be treated equally, could compete in sports, and become doctors and lawyers. Women could choose to do sports the same as men. We didn't have to rely on their fathers' or husbands' reputations. We didn't have to use their parents' money to go to college. We could get athletic scholarships. Women would be judged by their brains and physical abilities now and not just their pretty hair and boobs. Great. The world was changing. As a child, I thought anything I wanted was available to me.

After forty years, we haven't come that far. Our most admired and successful women are full of plastic surgery, got there because of their famous fathers or husbands, and still use sex instead of their brains to prove they are worthy of attention. But women in leadership is a topic for another book, so let me get back to the women who come to see me in their "middle age." My age group. As I publish this book, I am fifty-five. All pictures were taken when I was fifty-four. None of the pictures are photoshopped, and I have not had plastic surgery.

Today, most women work outside the home, raise the kids, and clean and care for the home. Compared to fifty years ago, more women work full-time jobs, and more women are doing it alone as single mothers. They are stressed all the time from lack of sleep and being constantly busy.

But our ideas of beauty haven't changed much. We still prize women for their physical attributes and want full busts, small waists and round butts, the classic hourglass figure. Women obtained this look through corsets in the 1800s, girdles in the 1950s, and now waist trainers. Just gross. To think we are beautiful by smashing our internal organs together is just painful and foolish. Please don't do that unless you want serious gastrointestinal and bladder problems. Women have come in wanting help with their gastrointestinal and bladder problems, not realizing why they have them.

Then we have the easier softer way to get the desired look. Plastic surgery. We get boob and butt implants and many different chemicals injected into our faces to fight off wrinkles, and facelifts starting at age forty. In South Korea, a country even worse than the United States for valuing beauty, on a girl's twenty-first birthday, she goes to get her first Botox injections with her mother.

Women do extreme diets to lose weight, like fasting or just eating meat and fat, and read whatever new diet book is out. This short-term weight loss is hard on the liver and kidneys and doesn't create the healthy body any woman is looking for in life.

The main thing I try to convince all women in this age group is balance. The balance between sleep, a good diet, exercise, and limiting stress. If we do these things, we can get the body we want internally and externally. None of these fixes come quickly, and a woman has to realize this will take a minimum of two years to get feeling healthy and make these long-term changes depending on where she starts.

Let's meet some women and see how they journeyed to a happier body and mind.

Martha was a forty-two-year-old woman with a litany of problems. Back hurts, aching joints, no strength, a history of asthma and infertility problems, probable chronic autoimmune disease. Always looked exhausted, didn't sleep well.

Martha always would put on a strained smile, trying to act like everything in life was great, the way she was taught to do as a woman. Women hold families together by doing multiple jobs and don't want to complain because there really isn't anyone to listen. Besides, they have so much to do, who has time to complain? Martha worked hard physically and stuck to it since day one with me. Now definitely my fittest client, she can do full-on pull-ups, push-ups, perfect sit-ups, sometimes I think she is fitter than me, almost!! Oh, and she looks great too. She truly is an inspiration to other women her age and her family. They have family CrossFit classes on Sundays in the garage. Beautiful.

Clare was a woman in her early forties when she started working out with me. In the beginning, she worked out with another woman. She had three kids and was very attractive, weight was good, but she wasn't fit or strong; in fact, she was kind of weak. She just looked soft and kind of sad. For her first few weeks, she would bring a bag she could throw up into just in case. Clare would get nauseous every time she worked out for about a month but never actually threw up. I always try to stop my clients before they lose their stomachs. It just doesn't get them to want to continue working out if it makes them throw up. Usually clients feel nauseous because their heart rate gets too high and they aren't used to this high heart rate. The heart starts pumping blood to the muscles and stops blood flow to the digestive tract. This is why a heart rate monitoring watch aids my job so much. I have enough experience to see it before it happens and slow a client down, but it affirms the high heart rate to the client, so they can begin to monitor the heart rate themselves and understand their cardiovascular abilities.

As she got fitter, she wanted to know where I thought she should be with her body and fitness levels. She showed me the picture of a model in a magazine and said, "I want legs that look like that."

"Great, I have to get you to one hundred twenty-five pounds, and you have to start running." She wanted the long lean thigh look. She thought that was too thin, and she couldn't even imagine running.

Clare started running slowly, slower than she ever dreamed of. I have new running clients learn how their hearts work and don't allow them to run over one hundred fifty heartbeats per minute for many months. At one hundred fifty beats per minute, they must walk until their heart rates are down to one hundred thirty beats per minute or less, and then they can start running again. This can be as slow as a fourteen- to fifteen-minute mile. We should not focus on the time of the mile but the result: getting fit. This is the same if the client is a kid or an adult. This woman had never been athletic sport-wise, but she had been into ballet as a child. Clare had no cardiovascular strength but was willing to do my go-slow running technique. It took almost three years, but she can now run very comfortably two to three days a week, keeping her heart rate under one hundred forty-five. She does 5Ks and 10Ks with her family, and her weight is one hundred twenty-five pounds. She has the body she has always dreamed of and didn't really think was possible. Her entire family is very fit, and they are that cute family you see at the Thanksgiving Turkey Trot. Yeah, Clare looks pretty hot as a woman in her late forties after having three kids and can rock a bikini on her Hawaiian vacation!

Liz had just moved to the area because her husband got a very high-paying job here. (I live in Silicon Valley). She had retired from the banking business and had big travel plans with lots of hiking planned so she needed to get fit, she told me. The vacations would involve over five miles a day of serious hiking. Liz had never worked out consistently before coming to me.

Liz is a great example of the changes in women's bodies we have seen in the last twenty or so years. Liz had a large hard belly that stuck out over her hips, extending about eight inches. The same beer belly look we always associated with men. Hard belly fat. She was very nice and worked very hard but was not willing to alter her eating habits. She would have a good week with food, cutting out carbohydrates and alcohol, then a bad week of eating out and drinking too much and go backwards with her weight and fitness. As much as I liked her, we just weren't getting anywhere after working out for about a year, so we parted ways. Liz looked about the same when she quit as when she started with me. She was just a little stronger. I was sad and felt I had failed to motivate her to want to lose that belly fat. Women like this worry me because they are walking heart attacks and strokes waiting to happen. I hope she is ok.

Beth's son hired me to work with her. Beth was seventy, retired, and had just lost her husband, the man's father, to a stroke. Beth was overweight, suffering from depression, and needed to exercise. Her son was very worried about her.

My first impression of her was that sadness had overwhelmed her with the loss of her husband. Beth was distraught with taking care of the family finances and was physically a mess. She was about fifty pounds overweight and had a litany of pains and excuses. She had already replaced both knees, but that didn't convince her she needed to work those legs to get muscle tone or take off the weight. She used marijuana and wine often to escape the pains of life.

Beth needed a why, and I was lucky to keep pressing until I found it. Her older dog had passed away in our first six months of working out together, and I helped her get Maggie, her cute little rescue dog from our local SPCA. Maggie is the center of her life and has come to the fitness studio many times to watch her mom work out. Hey, everyone knows I can't give up on a dog lover!

I really liked her, but her dedication was hot and cold. Beth knew she should be doing this exercise stuff, but showing up routinely was difficult for her. She consistently drank water and felt a whole lot better, and the weight was coming off slowly. She would tell me she felt better when she got in at least two workouts a week. She drifted away from working out with me after a vacation. I hope she is doing well.

I am not a fan of gastric bypass or any surgery that alters your stomach for weight loss. I had a client put the temporary balloon into her stomach, and that was a painful disaster: nine pounds of weight loss in one month and twelve pounds gained back after the balloon was removed.

I also am not a fan at all of weight-loss drugs and am shocked in 2021 that doctors still give out uppers for women to lose weight. These surgeries and/or prescription pills have lifelong effects that make living a regular life difficult. And if you did the surgery or took the pills but didn't change your lifestyle by adding diet and exercise—well, I have seen more clients gain the weight back or not get to a healthy weight after these surgeries.

I suggest you try diet and exercise first. Try it before resorting to surgery, thinking this is the easier way to weight loss. Your body will thank you later.

Marie came to me so excited when she moved back in with her parents. I was right around the corner—she could walk to me! She worked in the medical field and was very smart and very motivated. She had gastric bypass surgery and had lost about seventy pounds and needed to lose about forty pounds more to get to a normal body weight. She had pictures from ten years earlier when she was a very fit attractive woman. She now had had very thin arms and legs with all her excess weight still being around her midsection. She had worked out with many personal trainers, hated cardio, and loved lifting big weights. She wanted to do three workouts per week.

Marie was very high nervous energy. Always moving, always talking, and a very nice person but easily distracted. I had to keep her moving quickly from exercise to exercise. Marie did well at first and even started to do some cardio, though she initially hated it.

I had her running a full mile on the treadmill in eleven minutes without stopping for the first time in her life. The joy she had in doing this first mile quickly was amazing. She just beamed. But I could tell after six months we weren't really getting anywhere. Yes, Marie was stronger and felt better, but the weight wasn't coming off. She had to take sleeping pills every night just to get four hours of sleep in, gave up drinking alcohol for months at a time, and claimed to barely eat, drinking lots of water. Sometimes with overweight people, their metabolisms slow down so much that eating more than eight hundred calories a day causes them to gain weight. Lack of sleep is also a big factor in weight gain. She quit working out with me in less than a year. I hope one of these days Marie gets the body she deserves, with or without me.

Lisa walked in with the largest breasts I had ever seen on a normal-sized woman. She was 5'6" and about one hundred forty pounds with breasts that were easily triple F. These breasts came out of her tank top and up to her chin. She also had that weird flat stomach that is a sign of liposuction.

Her hair was bleached platinum, and her face was bumpy because it was so full of chemical injections. She came in because, "I want to get toned arms." She claimed to be a grandmother who didn't ever work a real job and was fifty-two years old. Lisa said she had a man who loved her and took care of her financially.

Lisa wanted two sessions a week. I doubted she would ever do two sessions in total with me. After her first session, when she was walking out, my next client, a guy, was walking in and said, "Is she a former porn star? Should I know her?" I was speechless. I just saw a woman who needed help. I hadn't even considered that was her former profession. And if it was, I didn't care. I just saw a woman who had gone to extremes to look a certain way, and I doubted I could help her. Her plastic surgery had damaged her body too much.

On her second appointment, Lisa told me she had breast reduction twice, so that is why she had all the scars in her armpits. I knew this was a lie because when she moved her left arm up over her head, her breast implant would pop up and almost touch her chin. Her breast implant had been put under her pectoral muscle, but something was wrong. It often would move, and she would push it back in place. I just smiled and tried to be accepting. Because of her breast implants, the connection of her pectoral muscles didn't connect with her biceps, so bench pressing or any exercise that activated her chest muscles was out of the question. Her main focus was her arms. She said she ran seven miles a day, but this was obviously a lie. She couldn't do cardio for more than five minutes because she couldn't breathe with the weight of the breast implants.

On her third visit, Lisa came in with even more injections in her face with it badly bruised. Her face was so full of fillers that her eyes were almost completely closed. She said she was "just puffy." It was all weird and uncomfortable for me. Then one day, Lisa just disappeared. She had paid for a workout, didn't come, didn't call, and didn't come back. I was super sorry that women felt they had to do this to their bodies to feel attractive. She had inflicted long-term damage on her muscles and bone structure to "look attractive" to someone. I was glad she quit; it was painful for me to watch.

This category probably has the most diversity, but all these women are brought together with the same problems. Stress, wanting to look a certain way to please others, and overall body weakness. Let's see the programs I use to help them feel better about their bodies.

# CHAPTER 17

# HELPING WOMEN GET THE BODIES THEY WANT AND DESERVE

A t fifty-four, as I write this book, I am in the best shape of my life, physically and mentally. (I know, way too much about me, but the mental aspect of our lives dictates our physical health.) Women don't have to give up and just accept that their bodies aren't going to be as healthy as they were in their twenties. It takes serious commitment and scheduling to keep your body healthy.

Most women juggle many hats by the time they hit their forties: wife, mother, single mother, daughter of aging parents, career woman, ex-socialite, housekeeper, cook, chauffeur for the kids, and classroom volunteer. There is no argument here: women's lives have become overly full and complicated. In most American households, the female does most of the house management, and over fifty percent of women do this while still holding down a forty-hour-per-week job outside the home, leaving little time for self-care.

A commitment to movement is essential. Exhaustion is so prevalent in this age group. The first thing is to figure out what time of the day works best for their schedules and have them commit to exercising at least five days a week during this time. It doesn't have to be for a full hour; it can be half. Just add a brisk walk, jog, bike ride, stair walk, yoga class, or workout with me into their schedule. This has to become a priority in their lives for their body transformations to succeed. And this really does need to be a commitment at least half an hour, five times a week, so working out and moving their body become habits. Housework doesn't count!

I know this is repetitive but...water. Every age group needs to make water drinking a conscious decision. Thirty ounces in the morning and thirty ounces in the afternoon at a minimum. Watch the coffee drinking. Many women drink coffee through-out the day. I have one client that drinks an average of six cups a day and avoids water, thinking this is a good alternative. I got her to drink two bottles of water a day, which is huge for her at sixty-eight and a major change. She knows she feels better drinking the water and that it helps her avoid the kidney stones she has had problems with for years.

Eight hours of sleep is always the goal, but seven hours will do with at least one and a half hours of deep sleep. This sleep needs to be uninterrupted as much as possible. Avoid alcohol before bed or large meals, especially meals with red meat. Both of these make the body focus on digestion or the liver work on getting rid of the alcohol, so the body can't properly relax for sleep. If you are having hormone problems, please see a doctor. Don't just struggle through menopause.

Okay, let's talk about how a woman's workout with me is different than a man's. Women have a slighter bone structure, don't develop as large or strong muscles, run slower due to their hip structure, and have a higher degree of body fat than men. These are just medical facts. I always laugh when a woman tells me she wants to be toned but not develop huge muscles. I have worked out consistently for over forty years and still don't have overly large muscles even when I was doing competitive weight lifting. It is very difficult for women to get large muscles without steroids, but all women can lower their body fat, get stronger, and get toned.

We raise boys and girls differently. My female clients in their late sixties or older never did sports as children. They tell me their mothers had them pick up sticks or jacks, play the piano, and do dance or ballet. They would never just go out in the yard and run around or throw balls. Most of them never learned how to throw or catch a ball and never developed eye-hand coordination. Most of my female clients never tried walking across a board between two chairs or other such dangerous kinds of things that would have helped them develop balance. Most boys did these kinds of things, fell, and tried again.

Sweating was just not allowed and considered gross, so these women avoided physical exertion their whole lives. I can't tell you how many women have walked into my studio telling me they don't sweat and are proud of this instead of realizing that not sweating isn't healthy. Sweating is how our body cools down. I get them sweating within ten minutes. If they are not sweating, it is because they are seriously dehydrated.

Because I mostly work with my clients, one on one, I can teach them how to throw a ball, run properly, and lift weights safely. If you are a woman and don't know these things, don't be embarrassed and definitely don't say, "I never wanted to learn to spiral a football." That's crap. I taught a sixty-five-year-old woman to throw a football, so she could play with her grandson when he came visiting for the holidays. I have never seen a woman so proud of herself after she got it. And being able to throw a football made her go home and want to practice even more. When we learn something correctly, we enjoy it and want to work at doing it even better. When we don't acknowledge that women want to learn how to use their bodies; we also deprive their minds from growing. Nobody just wakes up with sudden athleticism. It takes work and proper instruction.

The mind has to tell the body how to move so it all works together.

Women need to try many sports. Try tennis, basketball, golf, anything to get your body moving and that you enjoy. These will also be activities you can do with your significant other, family, and friends so you can now incorporate movement of the body into your weekly structure. We don't have to make food and alcohol our only reasons to be together with family or friends. Women love to be with other women, so I always encourage my female clients to make friends who they can enjoy playing sports with.

Women need to keep moving their bodies a priority for their entire lives. Don't put everyone else's needs in front of your own. Women are natural caretakers, but without taking care of your own mental and physical needs, there is nothing left to take care of others.

All women need to work on their strength, regardless of age. I have all women do a minimum of fifteen minutes a session of weight workouts. Strong bones and muscles will keep them going long in life with minimal pain. This strength also keeps a woman independent in life, so she can physically take care of herself.

Even my eighty-year-old clients need to jump a little. They can lean on something for security. The impact from jumping creates strong bones. Jumping also tightens up the lower muscles, aiding in a stronger bladder. Bladder problems are common in women, especially after childbirth. Many women come to me but are unable to work out for more than fifteen minutes without having to go to the bathroom. Within a year, they can do the full hour—run, laugh, everything—without having to worry about their bladders anymore or having accidents.

Exercise and good food habits can make strong women who feel happy in their bodies. Just find the exercise you enjoy and make it a priority.

# CHAPTER 18

# TEENAGERS, ATHLETIC AND NOT
## *THINK FITNESS, NOT SPORTS*

I get true joy from working with all of my clients, but this category is truly special for so many reasons to me. For me personally, I came into my personality from thirteen to fourteen years of age and incorporated my body and mind, working together into happiness. This is the age I stopped using food to fix me and found joy in running and started getting A's in school.

I am also very real in these chapters—not just about my "kids," or the kids I work with, but also about my own personal struggles as a teenager.

A Catholic priest pushed me in this direction and many others prodded me to continue heathier lifestyle choices, both physically and mentally. I definitely didn't always take these directions in the moment, but they always gave me something to think about, and I eventually took the advice of many people and still do.

Neither of my parents were physically or mentally well. Both were heavy drinkers, and my father was a serious smoker. Life problems were never discussed in my family. Emotions were not considered important. My brother started going to jail at the age of fourteen and never stayed out of jail for more than a year and a half, which he did while working for me when I was an organic farmer. My brother spent the majority of his life incarcerated. My sister graduated college by nineteen and worked very hard in an unhappy marriage until she died in her forties in a car accident. My brother was twelve years older than me, my sister fourteen years older than me. I was the product of an affair by my mother.

Even though I didn't know about the affair or why I was so different than my family from a young age, I didn't get along well with any of them, so the sense of "family" wasn't something I understood. At twenty-nine, I found out from my mother that I probably had a different biological father while she was dying from cancer. A DNA test later proved this, and after hiring a private detective to follow a man around, I got the DNA from my real father. He never knew I existed, and because he has a family, wife and two boys, I never chose to tell him. I didn't see the point in upsetting his life. He didn't leave me intentionally. He didn't know.

Even at a young age, I would try to have intellectual conversations about thoughts and feelings with my family. No family member would understand or participate. I spent my teenage years in books and plans of getting out of that family, which I did the day after high school graduation. But two suicide attempts happened first.

My first suicide attempt was at age eleven. I was fat, had no friends, and was a C student in school, and my parents were broke and drank heavily. I went out to a riverbed area in the city I grew up in. I crawled to the top of the ridge to jump off and die. I slid off the ridge and fell in soft sand, just getting a concussion and a broken leg. I hobbled home and went to work. I started doing things for money, cleaning horse stalls. I saved this money to buy a real home and get out of that mobile home we lived in.

At fourteen, in high school, I was trying to do it all. I was trying to party with my new friends, get straight A's, do sports, train for a marathon, date, work full time to pay the mortgage on the new home I had bought my mom, and just fit in. I slept four hours a night. I didn't think any of it was worth it. The rich people in town—I grew up in a small town where everyone knew everyone—still thought of me as less than because my dad was a deadbeat. I could never escape who my father was, no matter how hard I worked. I didn't have any brothers or sisters to guide me, and my mom was an alcoholic. I discovered the joy of cocaine. One night I was very depressed and tired, so I tried to snort enough cocaine to kill myself. Close to a heart attack, I was kept from falling unconscious by my drug dealer boyfriend until we got to the hospital. I lived. He dumped me the next week. I cleaned up my act.

All of this makes me an open book to all teenagers I work with and their parents. I always tell the teenager they can tell me anything. Nothing will shock me, nothing will make me think bad of them, and I will always answer every question with honesty. Mostly I just listen. Hormones are raging, and mental pain is common with this group, and most of it is stuffed down in frustration. Tears happen often in these conversations. We all need someone to listen to us. I try to be that person for my teenagers. I love them all.

Just like obesity runs in families, lack of physical activity runs in families. When a parent brings a child to me who is obese, it is because the family tends to be sedentary. This is not a family that plays tennis on the weekends and hikes seven miles on a Saturday or plays football on Thanksgiving. This is a family with TVs, teenagers with too much time alone, and parents who say, "Well, I am busy and not sports inclined, but I want my child to be different."

These are not families that cook together. I encourage families to make meals together. This encourages the use of real food and developing skills that will follow the child through their whole lives. Cooking together also gives families time for conversations.

When both parents are working over sixty-hour workweeks, the kids do school and nine extra-curricular activities and barely sleep because they have to Snapchat their friends, because god forbid they see their friends in person, this makes stressed-out kids who develop poor eating habits and lack of physical activity. As a family try to make at least make one meal together, like Sunday breakfast.

I have worked with male and female teenagers, athletic and not athletic. Some had pushy parents, and some were self-motivated. Some teenagers were very sad for many reasons. Teenage years are rough on everyone. I hoped to help these teenagers make it through those years just a little easier. Nothing makes me happier than watching these kids grow up to be young productive happy adults. And no matter their age, they will always be referred to as "one of Vanessa's kids."

I have to admit; this kid will be one of my favorites for my whole life. He calls me his best friend. All of the other kids know he is my favorite—sorry, I try to be impartial, but heck, I am human.

His father knew me from local running races. His father was in my same age group, nice man, decent runner, pleasant, lived close to me, and on long runs we would see each other and wave. We had never had more than a "hi" conversation, but he knew I was a personal trainer and that I was a high school coach.

His son, Adam was thirteen. Adam was kind of geeky according to his father. He had never been overweight or sports-minded. Adam would run with his dad on the weekends but never found a sport he was really interested in even though his parents had given him every opportunity to try everything from kid's soccer, tennis, even summer basketball camps. Nothing stuck or interested Adam. His father thought it would be good for his son to do cross-country in high school since it was a no-cut sport and his son already ran some with him. Could I maybe give his son some direction or a training plan for the summer to get ready for high school cross-country? "Sure," I said, "I would be happy to help Adam."

Adam was nice but not a kid in school you would notice. We ran five miles on the first time together, which was easy for him at about an eleven-minute pace, chatting the whole time. I liked him. I told him we would meet once a week, so I could work on running form with him, maybe do a longer run with him, and would monitor his runs on his Garmin watch. Nothing bothered this kid. He was very emotionally balanced and willing to work but not looking for any kind of greatness in sports. We laughed; we talked of his gangly legs, his need for more and more food. His mom worked very hard to keep Adam's weight up the more he ran. His sister rode her bike alongside of him and carried his water. Very loving supportive family. After ten weeks of training, he was solidly running forty miles a week, and I thought he was enjoying it. We did some sprint work the last week, but not a lot. I had put a solid base on him to get him to high school cross-country, but I didn't think much of it. Adam was just going to be one of the team. That is all he seemed to want to be. He never was the "cool" kid and didn't seem to want to excel at running. I just wanted him to be prepared.

High school started, and he tried out for the cross-country team at a good public high school. He was easily the best freshman, but not good enough for the varsity team. Because he had a strong base, I switched out the running workouts to do more interval work. Adam thrived running with the team and loved hanging out with the boys on the team. The first race came, and Adam easily won the junior varsity race. I wanted him on varsity; I felt he deserved it. The high school coach knew who I was when I walked up to talk to him and before I could speak said to me, "I don't put freshman on varsity unless they are exceptional." As a high school coach also at another school, I had to respect this even though it pissed me off.

The next day Adam and I went on a casual five-mile run. He looked at me and said, "I am tired of no one noticing me, I am just always not good, not bad. Just there, no one really notices me." This was more emotion than he had ever had in four months with me. We stopped running. He was crying, "Vanessa, why does no one think I can be good at anything?"

"I don't know. Why do you give a shit what everyone thinks? How about we show them?" was my response. The training kicked up.

The second cross-country race came the following week. Adam finished two minutes ahead of every junior varsity racer and would have been middle of the pack in the varsity race with his time. I just glared at the coach. Parents who didn't even know who I was knew I was pissed. The coach could no longer deny Adam was a good runner and agreed to make him part of the varsity team for the next race, only just to see how he would do in one race. No guarantees he would get to stay on the varsity team, the coach said to us as he glared at me. My mind kept saying, *All he needs is a shot. All anyone ever needs is a shot.* Ok, I will admit it, I wanted the shot to show Adam wasn't just a good runner, but a racer.

I beat into my Adam's head the next week that racing is different. We train at certain speeds, at certain distances, but racing is against others, and now we race. This would be the first time we had other runners in a race who were better than him, and I wanted him to be over-prepared. We practiced on the course. We talked about how Adam would position himself. This was a whole new thing. This was a race against kids who already had college scholarships and wanted to teach the fast freshman a lesson. Cross country can be brutal, mud splashed intentionally, blocking of your feet, elbowing. All this happens during cross-country races where the parents and coaches can't see. I told Adam to stay in fourth place, just working on being on the outside to the right within nine feet of the leaders as much as he could until mile two. Just work on even breathing and staying calm. The minute before he went to line up, I covered his watch with Duct Tape, so he couldn't look at it. Adam went to line up for the race, I went to the bathroom to throw up. His parents were both there, very excited to see their son race with the varsity team. His little sister was beyond excited, kept jumping up and down and grabbing my hand. I had pangs of jealousy, wishing I had a supportive family like that. *This isn't about you, Vanessa, this is about Adam,* I told myself as I tried to keep my stomach down. Adam glanced at me once and smiled and then the race took off. We wouldn't see Adam for about seventeen minutes. I followed him live on his Garmin watch.

His pace was super fast, about 5:20 a mile, and was even better than I expected. His heart rate was good, so his breathing was right on. As the racers started to come in, we saw number one and number two way ahead of everyone, about a minute. Then we could see a pack of four or so lightly dispersed runners in the distance. And there was Adam, smiling and pushing his stride to the largest I had ever seen him do, and finishing a solid third, racing so hard at the end. His high school coach smacked him on the back, his other teammate who finished in front of him hugged him, his parents screamed. I sat on the grass in awe; he looked at me and smiled and started to walk over. I told him, "No, you encourage your other teammates as they finish the race." I was crying. Adam was no longer the kid no one noticed. He had learned he could push himself beyond his ability.

He broke a five-minute mile in track his freshmen year and was the best cross-country runner in his league as a sophomore. Adam was offered a full ride high school scholarship at a prestigious boarding school back East. I encouraged him to take the scholarship even though he would leave me and his family for most of the year. This was far better coaching than I could give him, running with the top athletes in the country along with an amazing education. He went to the school and flourished as a runner and a student there, getting to 4:12 in the mile and landing a great college scholarship. He has great friends and a solid head on his shoulders. Even though he is away at college, we still talk every week. He will always be known as "one of my boys." To me, this is what high school sports, music, etc. can teach a teenager: that if they work hard and put their mind to something, they can have it. This is always the message I think sports should do for people. Teach them about hard work so it can cross over to the rest of their lives.

People always ask me when I knew Adam had the ability to be a top runner. I never knew that or expected it. All I knew was Adam was a kid who wanted to try hard and was willing to put in the work. I don't really hope I taught him to be a good runner. I hope I taught him to be a good person.

Angela's parents had worked out with me for a year or so, and their daughter was overweight and sad. After a suicide attempt at sixteen, her parents agreed to let me work with her. Actually, I begged them to let me work with her. I had worked out two other suicidal teenagers and felt I had something to offer Angela. I hoped the joy of exercise would help her brain as it had helped me as a teenager. She was not athletic, but I convinced her she could run a 5K in October and a 10K in November. She walked/jogged every day when she wasn't working out with me. The smile on her face when she finished those races was priceless.

She loves her shirts and her medals. Now she is thin, beautiful, and thriving in college with exercise and good food being a solid part of her life.

I had been the first female varsity coach of a boy's high school team in Northern California. I coached the tennis team for four years. There had been women coaching junior varsity boys but not varsity boys in many sports in Northern California. The other male coaches were downright mean and cruel to me. These fellow male coaches told me the wrong time for meetings, changed rules during matches, and were openly condescending to my boys and myself during matches. I was confused at this unprofessionalism in the beginning. Then I got angry when another coach started yelling at a player of mine. I took this coach's head off in public at the match then reported him to his principal on the phone right in front of him. I became my tennis team's hero at that point. I stood up for them and showed them how to take charge. I took a losing high school team in previous years to winning the league and making the playoffs every year since the first year I took over. In my first year as the Varsity Tennis Coach, I cut most of the seniors and had mostly all freshmen and sophomores on my team. We all established a special bond, and those boys were such an inspiration to me in learning how to coach teenagers.

I don't leave my phone ringer on in the evenings, usually. For whatever reason, I did that evening. At 9:30 p.m. one of the kids called. Ken didn't say anything; his end sounded more like a hiccup and lots of traffic. I yelled at him to tell me where he was.

Ken was up on a bridge off a freeway, threatening to jump off and kill himself. I tore out of my house and drove there. Police cars were surrounding him as he dangled off the overpass. I drove up and jumped out of my car, screaming, "Get the fuck down from there. You die and all of us live with it forever! How dare you?! Stop being so damned selfish!" A police officer grabbed me and pushed me away, throwing me to the ground. Ken came down from the chain-link fence and said, "Don't you dare touch coach!" He fell into my arms, crying and saying he was sorry. Ken lived with me for three weeks after that. His parents had been very pushy for him to succeed in school and tennis, and he had developed an eating disorder. At that time, he was eating just sweet potatoes. The whole tennis team rallied behind him to be his friend and get the psychological help he needed. Ken worked the teen suicide hotline while he was in high school and in college. He found giving back and helping others made him happy. He is thriving now at college. He gave up crash diets to lose weight. For about three years he had extreme food choices. Fasting, just sweet potatoes, all meat, all diets that made his blood sugar spike and drop and did not help him lose weight or become physically what he wanted to be. We worked on better eating habits, better steady exercise habits, and meditation. He gave up high-level competitive tennis, concentrating on school and helping others. So proud of him.

Evan was a ten-year-old boy who was very swaybacked and over thirty pounds overweight. He also was very pale, obviously rarely going outside in the sun. (We live in California, the land of skin damage.) His mom brought him in to do a group workout with her. She had stopped by earlier in the day to schedule a workout for herself and asked if her son could just sit there while she worked out. I said no, he could work out at the same time with her.

I do many classes of two to three people where the people are doing different things. They came into the studio; Evan was shy and admitted he didn't ever exercise. He said he mostly hung out alone and played computer games. I smiled and said it was all ok with me. The woman didn't work out at all during the personal training session. Everything seemed too hard, and she would do this nervous giggle and stop every exercise I wanted her to do after less than ten seconds. She just kept looked at herself in my large mirror. She was at least forty pounds overweight and not the least bit attractive. She kept posing in front of the mirror, and I just didn't get it. I kept trying to steal her away from the mirror and have her concentrate on working out, to no avail. She had no interest in working out and said it really wasn't a big deal that her son, Evan, was overweight. Her husband was also overweight and wouldn't agree to a personal trainer for their son since the father was overweight also. Then she dropped the bombshell. Evan was adopted. She had adopted him as a baby. I got angry at her. She was more obsessed with her fat body, and she was an overweight unattractive person physically and mentally. She is the first client I have ever completely yelled at during a session. I was so angry with her treatment of Evan and felt this was real child abuse. She admitted giving him two candy bars on the drive to my studio before the workout. She laughed as she told me this. I screamed at her.

Evan kept working out the whole hour, being completely oblivious to the heated conversation his mother and I were having. He had a blast moving his body, and I kept him busy. I got paid for that one session only by the father after a very angry phone call. The father was mad, and the mother was there and didn't think his son needed any help losing weight.

Two weeks later I saw a face against the glass of my studio trying to look in. I have reflective covering on my windows for privacy. I walked outside and saw it was the ten-year-old boy, Evan. I had another client in with me, so I just waved to him. He waved back. I told him to wait for me, I would be done with the current client in a few minutes. At the end of my client's session, I went outside, and Evan was still sitting there. I invited him in, put him on the rowing machine. I asked if he was ok. He smiled, "Vanessa, this was fun, can you teach me how to play football?"

"Sure, I can," I replied. "Do you have a cell phone, so you can text me to see when I have an open slot to fit you into?" I asked.

He did not. Evan said his mother and father didn't like me. He would just come by the studio when he could sneak away from his parents after school. I was ok with that. He would wave and sit outside if I was with another client. I worked him out, he laughed, we talked about the different kinds of foods to eat which would make him feel better. Evan promised to try. He promised not to eat candy bars before coming to work out with me. Evan came to my studio weekly for about a month, then with no notice, he just stopped coming to the studio and disappeared.

I figured his parents found out and grounded him. I didn't charge his parents for any of these sessions that was just Evan.

A year later I saw his mother in the grocery store. She was thinner and had on tons of makeup. I was hoping she was buying healthier food options for her family. I stopped her and asked, "How is Evan?"

"Oh, we had to give him back," she said as she smiled and walked away.

"Wait!" I yelled, startling many shoppers around me. "What does that mean?"

"It means we were unfit parents and the adoption people took him back."

I cried for weeks after that. I should have stepped in and done something. I hope I see him again someday and that he found a better home.

A mother called me inquiring about her fourteen-year-old daughter. Her daughter had a heart condition that needed consistent exercise. I met Natasha with her mom. Natasha barely spoke during this first meeting and was about twenty pounds overweight and looked soft, like she rarely exercised, and was very shy. We started working out twice a week. I never had a client that constantly went to the hospital before. I think Natasha went to the hospital about once a month in the beginning. She would get massive amounts of morphine injected for the constant pain in her abdomen. Natasha had been sick since the age of eight, which caused her to miss school and most other extra-curricular activities. She always stuck with her workouts though and got healthier as she aged. She is now attending college and is a very strong smart woman. Great to watch her grow up.

These stories are a great example of different kinds of teenagers. Now let's look at how to get them motivated to move their bodies and eat healthier foods.

# CHAPTER 19

# LIFELONG MOVEMENT AND GOOD EATING HABITS FOR SOON-TO-BE ADULTS

Teenagers need to be constantly moving and talking. It's just where they are in life, whether they are doing athletics or just trying to get fit. I work this aspect into all of my activities with teenagers. Listen to them. Talk and encourage them to move while they do it.

With younger kids, nine to thirteen, I try to get them balanced and cardiovascular fit. This allows them to do any sport they choose as they grow up. Then I introduce them to hand-eye coordination. This gives them the basics to go forward in any direction.

If a child comes to me already competing in a sport like tennis, running, soccer, etc., the first thing to figure out is whether it is the child who wants to do the sport and compete or is it the parents pushing the child. I don't put up with pushy parents. This creates long-term damage to the child physically and mentally.

Karen played on my high school tennis team. Karen was fourteen years old, a freshman, and had been playing tennis for over six years with private instruction and was fairly good, not great. She was very timid but had good basic tennis skills. Karen was always talking badly about herself though, and I didn't get it. She was attractive, a good tennis player making varsity as a high school freshman, and an A student. She had friends. When I would do the lineups for actual matches, she would beg to not play. I made her play matches anyway, and Karen was constantly looking toward me for advice and played her tennis matches horribly, way under her ability. She would lose her matches most of the time and cry hysterically afterward.

I called her mother and demanded she come talk to me at the next day's practice. She had not come to see her daughter play her matches and didn't come to the parents meeting, so I hadn't met her. I made all the parents meet me personally and come watch at least one match that their children played in. This was a requirement for being on the team, parent participation. Karen was in hysterics that I was having this meeting with her mother. I didn't know if Karen had a father in her life; she never spoke of one, and I never asked.

The next day Karen's mother came to tennis practice. She was angry to have to be there and take off work to meet with me. The mother had a scowl on her face and her arms crossed. Karen wouldn't even look her mother in the eye, instead kept her head down and looked at her feet while she moved around uncomfortably. I thanked the mother for coming and explained to her that Karen was a good tennis player but didn't seem to like playing and definitely didn't like competing. In fact, Karen was very scared to compete and would sabotage herself into a loss. I asked the mother for insight into her daughter's behavior.

The mother grabbed her daughter's arm roughly shaking her and started yelling at her in another language so I couldn't hear what was said. I calmly told the mother to take her hand off her daughter on my tennis courts now or I would call the police. I told Karen to go and be with her friends who were all watching from a few feet away, all scared by what they were watching. I stayed very calm.

The mother went to walk away from me, and I told her if she walked away from me her daughter would be off the tennis team. The mother came back seething. I told her I didn't care if Karen played tennis on the team. I cared if her daughter was mentally healthy. Karen's mother told me it was none of my business.

"Oh, that is where you are very wrong. If I find out you have physically abused your daughter, I will call Child Protective Services, as I am required to do by law, and you will be investigated. Twelve young girls are listening to this conversation, so you better watch yourself and how you treat your daughter from now on because you do anything bad to Karen, and I will know." I knew I was barely under control. I was physically shaking. The mother stormed off and all the girls came over to hug me. Karen was shaking and thanked me. I asked if there was anyone else she could live with, and she said no but she thought she would be ok and would let me know every day how she was doing.

Karen blossomed on the tennis team after I confronted her mother. She laughed, she won a couple of matches, she lost a couple of matches. She met a boy, she learned to code. Our tennis season ended and so did my communication with her on a daily or weekly basis.

Four months later I was with a personal training client, and my phone wouldn't stop ringing. The call was from the athletic director of the school. Karen was up on a bridge, wanting to jump. I was there in ten minutes.

The police had blocked off the bridge. A group of people were watching her, mostly students. The police let me through, and Karen came down and hugged me crying. "I just can't be good enough, Coach, I just can't be good enough."

I said nothing as we sat crying on the concrete bridge. This was my second child that had physically tried to commit suicide in front of me, and I was at a loss. Our expectations in life are so high we think this is the only answer. Suicide.

"Ah, that's ok. I am never good enough, let's go get ice cream."
Everyone parted out of our way, and we calmly walked to my car.
I avoided looking at her mother, and we went to get ice cream.
Social services went to her house that evening and set up a mon-
itoring program of the mother. Karen also has a younger brother.

I am very happy to say now Karen is in her second year at
USC. She comes and sees me on her school breaks just for that
ten-second hug. I had a client with me one day, and Karen said
to my client, "Sorry to interrupt you, I have to hug Vanessa, she
saved my life." My answer always is, "Nah, I just bought you
ice cream." I remind her that daily exercise helps fight off the
demons that bring on depression. She shows me her Fitbit.

Her mother became softer after the suicide attempt and explained
to me she was only trying to get her kids the best possible lives.
She bakes me things often. She is thankful I was in her daughter's
life and tries to be a better mother. We all make mistakes; we just
need to be open enough to learn from the mistakes and move on.

Sugar, fast food, and carbohydrates are mainstays of children
and teenage diets. These bad food decisions affect their brains
greatly with emotional spikes. I always try to get young adults
to eat better by making plans on how to eat. Teenagers need to
learn how to cook. This will be very important when they go off
to college.

I try to install in all of the kids I work with a love of their bodies
and what they can do with them. Sports and working out needs

to be playful and full of laughter. This will keep them happier and balanced.

Encourage children to make friends through sports even if they are just running around the yard. Encouraging children to choose physical activities at a young age can help them throughout their lives.

# CHAPTER 20

# OVER 70

## *"NEVER DONE IT," "IT'S TOO HARD," "MY BODY'S SHOT."*

N̲o other category has defined my career like people over the age of seventy. This is always the group of people I am most concerned about and work very hard to help. And the reason someone over seventy has called me—can't walk, arthritis, obesity, etc.—isn't the real problem with this age group. It is about the loneliness and isolation.

I didn't grow up with grandparents or other relatives, so I didn't even know people over the age of seventy before I started working as a personal trainer. When I first started getting clients in this group, the common denominator wasn't their physical state, but their mental state. I would never say that to them or the families that have hired me in the beginning of working together. Most of the people over seventy years of age were sedentary, watched TV most of the day, could barely walk or move without serious pain, took many medications, and thought all of this was a normal way to live at their age. Their friends had died, their spouses had died, and their children had moved away and had full lives that didn't involve their parents anymore. Boredom is common. Time just passes without doing much of anything physically or mentally. Consequently, their bodies break down from lack of movement until just getting out of a chair becomes difficult or impossible. Hence, they call me for help.

Common traits in men and women in this group are people that haven't exercised their entire lives or since they were children. The most common reasons I am called: they can no longer walk without pain, had a heart attack or stroke, or can't get out of a chair. I am usually hired by a family member.

I always make this group see a doctor and get a full battery of tests before we start working out together. This group of tests includes a full blood panel, a stress test, and an overall in-person physical.

Most people don't understand their medical records, especially their blood tests. People feel rushed in doctors' offices and try to ignore medical and physical problems in the hope the medical issue will go away or get better with time. I go through the medical records and tests with them, giving them notes and questions to take back to the doctors. I teach them to look at the history of their tests and understand the changes. I especially want them to understand their blood pressure.

No other group tells me "I can't," "It is too difficult," or "I don't like this" more often. Even a little jog in place can set them off into a negative spin. I try with this group to move very slowly and find the motivation. Is it walking, is it improving their golf games, playing with their grandchildren, just getting into and out of a car comfortably, being able to shop alone? Find the motivation and give them exercises toward making that goal possible and painless.

I didn't learn overnight how to take care of people over seventy. In the beginning I would say, "You know many people your age run marathons or golf every day; you just have to get moving." Then the clients would feel bad and get negative and tell me that wasn't normal people for their age and I was talking about the exceptions. All of their friends were in worse physical shape and this comparison didn't motivate them as it did younger age groups. I stopped speaking this way. I realized I was bringing guilt and negativity into their lives and I had to do it differently. I focus with them on positively getting better than they were before they met me. Let them ask me if they can move forward to a sport or greater physical activity. Not me pushing them.

Let's meet some of these amazing adopted grandparents of mine and let me show you how they changed not just their lives but my own.

Allison was seventy-two when she called me and was having trouble walking. She was a lawyer, still working part-time. She had been a fairly famous lawyer in my area, arguing in front of the Supreme Court, and a trailblazer as a female lawyer in the 1970s. Allison had tried a group workout place for a while, liked it, and felt it helped her, but the gym closed down.

Her office downtown was about two blocks from the courthouse. One day she was walking to the courthouse, and just carrying her briefcase and walking for those two blocks was almost too much. She stopped to rest, and a younger lawyer in her office offered to carry her bag. She was embarrassed and called me to see if I could help her physically, so she could get around easier.

One of the first things Allison said to me was, "I am an energy conserver." She didn't like exercise, never wanted to exercise in her life, had gastric problems, was about twenty-five pounds overweight, and very weak looking I thought for her age. Allison was proud to tell me she never broke a sweat.

I always find this hysterical and a weird thing to be proud of, so much that you would want to share this information with a personal trainer. Because many people over seventy have said this to me, I began to realize how sedentary this age group had become. *How can someone be proud of never using their bodies to their full potential* had always been my thought.

For the first time in her life, I got Allison to sweat every time she saw me. She didn't think she could. Not drinking water was a bad habit of hers, and it took us over five years just for her to get two glasses of water down a day. I don't push her hard and never set her up to fail. Allison also has no attention span for paying attention to or moving her body. I leave it all alone and just work her out as much as she can. We are working on breathing which doesn't come naturally to her, and I don't argue with her. Any movement she does with me is better than the nothing she used to do by herself, and I accept that.

Discovering podcasts she loved was the trick to get her to walk by herself once I had made her strong enough. She will only allow herself to listen to her podcasts when she walks. This listening to podcasts is the enticement to get her out of the house and walking. Always have to find a way to help a person want to better their bodies. Allison walks about six miles a week and works out with me twice a week.

I don't bug her about the weight which has never come off. She is much stronger now eight years later and much healthier than when we started. That is more than enough.

I got a phone call from an older man asking if I could go into a residential facility and work out his daughter. I was slightly confused, then a woman also began to speak on the phone. She said her daughter had taken a fall, didn't have any insurance, and was in a Medicare facility that didn't provide any physical therapy. I listened to both of their voices and was still very confused. They said their daughter was seventy years old. The parents were ninety and ninety-one. I agreed to meet their daughter and see what I could do.

I had been in retirement facilities many times but very upscale expensive ones. This was my first time in a Medicare facility, and it was horrible. The smell, the cheap furniture, the people who looked like zombies just sitting in wheelchairs in the hallway. I didn't know if I could do it. I talked to the administrator and signed the release allowing me to work with Martha. I went to her room to meet her.

She was frail. She had broken her back after a suicide attempt in her barn. She couldn't walk and was scared of everything. She was frantic. We worked on breathing exercises, and I showed her how to move her body. I saw her three times a week. It took me two months to get her to stand up. Every time she said she couldn't do it, I reminded her I needed to get her walking so she could go home. In month three, she began to walk around her room with a walker. The first time Martha walked down the hall with her walker and waved to the employees, she smiled. After that first walk, I couldn't stop her. She wanted to walk on her walker for an hour a day. After six months, she left the facility and went home. She is now seventy-four and doing great.

In the front of this book, I made a dedication to a very special man, Jack. Jack is the only client's real first name I use in this book. This man really started off my journey as a personal trainer and showed me I could actually help people. I loved Jack so much. He has since passed away, but we had fun for a number of years. I hope you enjoy meeting him and that my words can express the joy I had working with him.

His daughter hired me. She lived in a different state and Jack lived in a retirement community. Jack was eighty-five and in a motorized wheelchair. His daughter didn't know why he began to use this motorized wheelchair all the time. He had a nice one-bedroom apartment in a retirement village. He would go down to the community area for breakfast, lunch, and dinner. I figured 10:00 a.m. would be a good time for me to work out with him.

The daughter who hired me warned me he watched Fox News all day and was grouchy. She had a brother who lived in the San Jose area and would meet me at the retirement village the first time to do introductions with his father. The daughter was very hopeful I could help her dad. She knew her dad was deteriorating quickly from the lack of physical activity.

His son met me in the parking lot. He was uncomfortable introducing me to his father. The son kept saying his father was grouchy and wouldn't want to work out with me. When we went into the apartment, Jack barely looked up. His son explained that I would be coming to work out with him a couple of times a week, and maybe he could be nice to me. Jack was disinterested in me being there. He was more interested in whatever was on Fox News. I explained to the son I was fine, he could leave.

Jack didn't want me there. He was not going to be polite. He complained about his heart condition, the fact that his legs didn't move because he had neuropathy. He told me his joints had worn out since he had been such a big man at over 6′4″ and about two hundred forty pounds. I was patient and listened. I had him move his arms a little, got those legs moving, and got him out of the chair onto his walker. Jack tolerated me on that first meeting. In the beginning, I saw him twice a week.

But I got Jack talking and moving. I distracted Jack by asking him about his wife. He loved her so much and she had passed away five years earlier. After his wife died, his family decided to move him into this retirement community. He would cry as he talked about his wife and the things they used to do. He could remember dinners they had in nice restaurants and the things she used to say to him. They had three children, one girl and two boys. He was close to his daughter and not to his boys. I would just keep him talking while making him move his body. Sometimes we would play basketball with a basketball and a trash can, sometimes soccer into a small net I would bring. Anything to get him moving and laughing. He told his daughter how much he enjoyed working out with me, and she asked me to come five days a week. I was delighted. I loved working with him and listening to him tell me about his life.

I had been with him for about two months. He could now get up out of his motorized wheelchair and onto his walker easily and walk around the apartment. Within six months I had him walking down the hallway and back for about five to ten minutes. He was happy now. He would laugh and tell me jokes and asked about my running or tennis tournaments. He laughed about my bad dates. Jack always wanted to see pictures of my dogs. I showed him how to use a computer. He had refused for years to use one and never wanted a smartphone. I put him on Facebook, so he could see the great-granddaughter he had never met that had recently been born.

He had a girlfriend that lived in the retirement village and would come over to his apartment when I was done with his workout. They would have meals and talk. His family didn't care for her intrusion. I liked her. She dressed up in fancy clothes and had lived a fascinating life. I could listen to her talk for hours too. I thought she was good for Jack.

I began to know all the staff, the housekeepers, and LVNs who passed out his medications. One day I got there, and the house-keepers were giggling, waiting outside his door for me to get there. I said, "What is going on?" They all laughed and said, "Nothing, Vanessa, go on in." I went in, said hello to Jack, then saw something on his carpet going into his bedroom.

"Jack, why are there black-lace panties on the floor? Why did you let her leave them there so the entire community would know the two of you had sex? She left her mark, so everyone would know."

"Vanessa, I can have sex with anyone I want, and you can't stop me! I am a grown man, I can do what I want, and it is none of your business," he told me in a huff.

"No, Jack, it isn't any of my business, and of course you can do what you want, but do you even know if you really had sex?" We both laughed our heads off. He walked even farther that day, zipping down the hallway. He began to drink a little wine with some guys in the evenings while they played cards after dinner. He was making friends and laughing. Some older ladies who hung out by the door when I would walk into the facility began to call me Jesus because I made Jack walk. His daughter came to visit as did some of his grandchildren. It was delightful. He was the first person I got out of a wheelchair and walking. I watched him blossom as a human being the more he moved his body.

When Jack had a birthday and turned eighty-six, I asked him if he had any wisdom he had gained in the past year he wanted to pass down to me. "Vanessa, stay out of the bars." We laughed. If only he had told me that forty years earlier, my life would have been so much better!!

One day I got to Jack's apartment, and the son I had never met was there with his wife. They lived about a six-hour drive away. They knew about me, and I offered to leave and come back in the afternoon so they could visit with Jack. I could feel the tension in the air. This was the son Jack had never gotten along with at all. They said, no, they were leaving, I could stay. He barely said goodbye to them as they walked out. As they shut the door, Jack was crying, "Vanessa, why does my son hate me, I tried to be a good father, we just didn't know how to talk back then, it wasn't my fault."

I dropped my bag and ran down the hall after his son. "Please don't leave. Your dad really wants to make it up to you. He is sorry you two don't like each other."

His son looked at me and said, "He likes you better than me, his own son. We will leave." They turned to walk away again, and well, never being one to keep my mouth shut, I yelled, "Asshole!"

The son turned around with anger, and before he could talk, I grabbed his arm and pulled him back into the apartment. He saw his dad crying. I left and came back a few hours later. They were still talking. Priceless.

In retirement communities, the administration is always nervous about the tenants being injured from falling and prefers to keep them in wheelchairs. I, of course, hated the wheelchairs which I felt made the people deteriorate even more from lack of movement and using their muscles. I would take Jack outside in his motorized wheelchair, and we would race in the parking lot. Once he was going as fast as he could in the motorized wheelchair, and he hit a speed bump in the road and "caught air" and almost crashed. I had to grab the chair before it turned over. It was hysterical. We laughed for weeks about it. The administration of the retirement community didn't like me, obviously.

Jack's hips began to fail as he aged, and his congestive heart failure was getting worse. I knew the end was near. He had to move into convalescent care the last few months of his life. I couldn't work with him there anymore—administration's rules. I would still go visit him, but it was so sad I would always leave crying. We treat humans at the end of their lives horribly. I wouldn't ever treat my dogs that badly.

I know putting our elderly in these kinds of homes sometimes is necessary because other family members can't physically or financially take care of them. But these homes are just places to go die, and they are very sad and lonely places.

I will always miss Jack who taught me patience and compassion and how to get people out of wheelchairs and walking. What I learned with him I have taken to many other clients.

# CHAPTER 21

# GETTING PEOPLE OVER 70 TO MOVE

nderstanding someone's limits and wants is very important in this age group. No group is more limited by their mental thoughts. Many of them are just too scared to move their bodies because they have never moved their bodies their entire lives. Any new kinds of activities or movements must be introduced slowly. Realize pain has become a regular part of their lives and try to relieve them of that pain as much as possible by showing them movement can actually help them. Movement reduces inflammation. Much of the pain in my elderly clients is caused by inflammation.

We have become a society that takes many prescription pills. I always try to get these clients to understand why they are taking the pills and work with their doctors to see if they can get off of them. Kidney damage from the long-term use of pills is common. Most clients don't know if it is their back causing pain or their kidneys.

Try to get any people in your life who are over seventy years of age into a social group. Isolation in this group is common, which brings depression and then even less movement. Walking is so important. Make sure they keep up their strength with weight work even if it is just small one-pound weights. Get them to stretch and move so their arms can still go straight. Have them understand that arthritis can be kept at bay when constant movement occurs.

Visit them. Don't leave older family members or acquaintances alone to die feeling unappreciated or unwanted. I saw too many people in the retirement communities I worked in that never had visitors and just stared at a TV all day. No one wants to live that life.

Make working out a game. I play basketball, soccer, catch—all kinds of games with my clients. This keeps them not just moving but working on eye-hand coordination.

# CHAPTER 22

# TAKE YOUR FIRST STEP

## *SET ACHIEVABLE GOALS*

know you expected a book of exercises and quick fixes on diets and Shangri La. Instead, you heard of suicides, depression, dating, and the realities of the human body. I wanted to express mentally what we need to do to make our bodies better and how interconnected the mental and physical aspects of our bodies are. Both need work to feel healthy.

I want you to find your happy place with your body, as many of my clients have, and realize this has to happen every day of your life. There is no quick fix and moving on to the next thing. This is daily good healthy self-care of your body and making decisions on how you want to live.

I make jokes all the time about why I run so much. But the truth is being fat caused me to be depressed and full of rage. Running saved my life as a thirteen-year-old and still does today forty years later. I run twenty to forty miles a week usually at 4:30 a.m. This puts my brain chemistry in the right balance, so I don't kill myself or others. And this is no joke: I have made three serious suicide attempts, obviously failing all times. The times I tried to commit suicide, I had stopped physically working out and had become bedridden with depression. We know physical activity can be as good as many psychiatric drugs, so encourage anyone you know who is having a difficult time to move their bodies. Don't just meet friends or family for a coffee or glass of wine. Meet them for a tennis match or a nice hike. Get sunshine. Vitamin D deficiency is very common in the winter months and aids the depression.

There are no quick fixes in life. All surgeries come with rehabilitation that must be done. Plastic surgeries to make you look better are temporary fixes. I have seen personal friends get liposuction and then gain even more weight back.

Set good short-term achievable goals. When a client walks in and says, "I want to lose forty pounds in two months," I usually laugh. There is no way to do that successfully and keep the weight off. Instead, I work with the client to be reasonable. "You didn't gain forty pounds in two months, so it isn't coming off in two months. Let's work on losing one pound a week and getting regular exercise, sleep, and nutrition." These are concrete doable actions. Achievable goals.

Be positive. Negativity gets us nowhere.

When life gets you down, as it will, fight against that want to go to unhealthy food, drugs, and alcohol as fixes. Go to what you know makes you feel better—moving your body in constructive ways through exercise and using food as nutrients and not to hurt you.

# CHAPTER 23

# STAY MOTIVATED FOR LIFE

Why do we live? What do you expect and want out of life? You and only you can figure out what will motivate you. Not all motivation is internal; some is external. The first step is taking the time to understand yourself. Are you a loner or someone who prefers to be in a group? Do you like a little bit of both?

In the beginning of this book, I started off by having you admit who you are now and what you want to do in life. We are all very different, as you have read from the chapters about all of my clients. Now is the time to put it all together.

Who do you want to be? Yeah, I know you laughed when your brother jokingly said that he didn't realize guys could get pregnant and asked, "How many months are you?" And it was so cute when your husband said, "Oh, but honey, it is cute when your butt fat wiggles." You smiled and nodded and laughed but hurt inside. You looked at those pictures of the models and sports stars in magazines and wondered, *Why are they lucky and I am not?*

But you can make your own luck through better eating habits and exercise. Take just that thought that you want to change. Take that one moment that you are thinking about changing and do something physical. For just that one moment, do three push-ups. Do three sit-ups. Walk around the yard. Jog twenty-three steps. Don't just think and wish, *do* for just that moment. And feel proud of yourself internally that this time you didn't just think, you *did*.

*It was a hard day at work and the kids are screaming. I think I will have a scotch. How about if I have a full glass of cold water first before the scotch? Then maybe some cucumber and tomato slices.* Meditate for two minutes with great deep breathing. Do you still want that scotch?

*Look at those grandkids. I want to watch them grow up to be amazing humans, graduate college, marry, laugh. Am I healthy now at sixty-five to be a thriving adult and someone they will want to be around at eighty-five? If not, what do I need to change to stay healthy as I age?*

What do your kids want more than anything? Someone to play and spend time with them. Can you physically and mentally be there for them, and if not, what do you need to change to make that happen?

Take a look at your family and friends. Are they living the healthy lifestyle you so crave? If not, how can you change your lifestyle so you are an example of healthy living? Can you make healthy dinners everyone wants? Can you enjoy activities that aren't focused around processed food, sugar, and alcohol?

Go to your local park. Watch strangers playing baseball, walking and playing with their dogs, kids throwing a Frisbee. Close your eyes and what do you hear? Laughter. Moving our bodies and playing sports with others creates laughter and happiness. Watch the end of a local 5K. See the smiles on the runners' faces who aren't racing to win the race, but moving their bodies and finding extreme joy. Put yourself out there by moving your body and grabbing some of that joy. Encourage your family and friends to do the same.

Keep those fat pants and those pictures of yourself where you are very overweight and/or unhealthy looking. Remind yourself of how unhappy you were with that extra weight that hurt your back and knees and kept you from interacting with others. Feel compassion for that person you used to be and remember the pain. Be proud of the new person you are as you move forward being healthier, loving, and taking of your body.

Be a constant student of yourself and your body. Learn to listen to yourself. Remember—*it's your body: move it, love it, live.*

# ACKNOWLEDGEMENTS

Thank you for reading my book, and I hope you found some inspiration on your fitness journey. This book happened because of the support and help of many people.

First, Ms. Perla Jimenez, my videographer, photographer, and social media manager in my San Jose, CA location. Thank you, Perla. Without you, this book would not have happened. Thank you for having the patience to make me look good when I was past the exhaustion level many times.

Next, thank you to all the clients of the past decade who have trusted me to help them on their fitness journey and taught me so much about patience, perseverance, and hope.

And finally, thank you to my mother, Julita, who passed away from undifferentiated cancer at the age of sixty-three when I was twenty-nine years old. She tried. Even though we didn't have any money and she worked full time so she didn't have much to spare, she always tried to give me everything she could and support me in any way possible. She had fried egg sandwiches ready for me at the end of every morning run when I was a kid, raced after work to show up to the last few minutes and watch me finish a cross country race in high school, was there when I ran my first marathon, was there when I won my first marathon, was there for every last place in my horse shows as a child, watched me win a Grand Prix horse jumping competition as an adult, saw me eat my first organic strawberry, and looked so sad for me after every broken relationship.

Mom, I love you and talk to you every day, when I win, and when I lose. I always think when a crow squawks at me, it's you talking to me. Thank you for showing me how to work hard and keep taking every opportunity life throws at me.

# ABOUT THE AUTHOR

Vanessa Bogenholm lives and works her truth every day, both in her own life and with each and every client. Some days, she would still rather be the unmotivated, overweight ten-year-old sitting on the couch eating candy, but she can't be. She can't because she wants better for herself and because she wants to show her clients—and you—that with a little belief and a shift in attitude, you don't have to be stuck in a body that makes you uncomfortable.

CPSIA information can be obtained
at www.ICGtesting.com
Printed in the USA
BVHW090246150921
616748BV00008B/639/J

9 781544 522616